UNDERGRADUATE OBSTETRICS AND GYNAECOLOGY

Undergraduate Obstetrics and Gynaecology

M G R Hull MB BS FRCOG
Gillian Turner MB BS FRCOG
D N Joyce MA DM MRCOG

Consultant Senior Lecturers
Department of Obstetrics and Gynaecology
University of Bristol

Edited by
G Dixon PhD MB BS FRCP FRCOG

Professor, Department of Obstetrics and Gynaecology
University of Bristol

Bristol
John Wright & Sons Ltd
1980

Published by John Wright & Sons Ltd., 42–44 Triangle West, Bristol BS8 1EX.

British Library Cataloguing in Publication Data

Hull, M G R
    Undergraduate obstetrics and gynaecology.
    1. Gynecology
    2. Obstetrics
    I. Turner, Gillian
    II. Joyce, D N   III. Dixon, Geoffrey
    618   RG101

ISBN 0 7236 0564 5

Printed in Great Britain by
John Wright & Sons Ltd. at the Stonebridge Press, Bristol BS4 5NU

Preface

The recent rash of curriculum changes which has broken out in almost every medical school in the UK has placed more and more stress on 'scientific medicine'. Students often find it difficult to appreciate the importance of their pre-clinical training as a preliminary to their entry into the clinical curriculum, and part of the aim of this book has been to emphasize some of the theoretical aspects of obstetrics and gynaecology and their relationship to other disciplines, especially endocrinology and psychiatry, as well, of course, as general medicine and general surgery.

There are a few who would favour the exclusion of the specialty in its traditional form from the undergraduate curriculum, making it entirely a postgraduate subject. We are opposed to any such suggestion, partly because in many cases the obstetrical course gives students their first direct introduction to patients and the opportunity to play some part in and take some responsibility for patient care. We also feel that whatever branch of medicine is finally adopted by the student he needs some background training in obstetrics and gynaecology. However, since anybody who is to undertake practical obstetrics and gynaecology either as a specialty or as part of general practice has to undertake postgraduate training we have deliberately omitted much specialized detail from the work. A notable absentee is the customary chapter on history taking and examination of the gynaecological patient. These are subjects which can only be learnt in contact with patients, whether it be in the wards or in clinics. A further motivation for the omission was that in these days of rapidly rising book costs the inclusion of a chapter which will only be read once during the student's career is unwarranted. Equally, both student and reviewer will search in vain for the usual chapter on operative gynaecology. Again, this omission is deliberate because we do not feel that an intimate knowledge of operative detail is part of the present-day student's ambit. While the main purpose of an undergraduate's attendance in an operating theatre is to learn to glean the correct information from pelvic examinations, they do inevitably receive sufficient basic information to be able to explain to patients the necessity for and the results of major gynaecological procedures. Also we must draw attention to the fact that we have omitted many details of neonatal management. We have taken this step because paediatricians should instruct the undergraduates in neonatal resuscitation and the recognition of the normal and abnormal baby and its management. We feel sure that every student should be in possession of a suitable text dealing with the neonate and its problems.

In attempting to write an extremely concise book which covers both branches of the specialty and the relation of clinical practice to the basic knowledge of anatomy, physiology, biochemistry and pathology, we have inevitably been forced into colouring black or white some areas which in a less concise book would be grey. Once again this is a deliberate policy adopted in the hope that it may avoid or diminish some of the heart-searching perplexity which the modern student may experience. In this book we have attempted a rational approach which we hope will be used to complement bedside and clinical teaching and any system of tutorials and lectures which are adopted in individual hospitals.

All sections have been read by all the authors and have often been the subject of lively discussion and debate. Nevertheless, we have not tried to become uniform in either our opinions or our writing styles, although we have, as has been stated, coloured our subjects black or white rather than grey. We felt that any effort at studied uniformity would result in a lifeless book which would give little pleasure to the students or their instructors.

Without the combined and industrious efforts of Mrs J. Davies, Mrs W Cann, Mrs A. Coles and Mrs C. Saunders, our departmental secretaries, this book would not have appeared. We are extremely grateful to them all for their great help. The illustrations are the work of Miss H. Field and to her we also express our gratitude. Finally we would wish to thank Dr J. A. Gillman and his colleagues at John Wright & Sons Ltd for their forbearance and patience at the delays that have occurred when the pressure of clinical work has made our more academic pursuits not only difficult but at times impossible.

October 1980   G.D.
                                                                                 D.J.
                                                                                 M.H.
                                                                                 G.T.

Contents

Chapter one

Reproductive Physiology

Introductory Note: Gestational, Embryonal and Fetal Age

The distinction between gestational age and embryonal or fetal age needs to be carefully made when considering events in early pregnancy relating to embryological development. In this book, being clinically orientated, gestational age will invariably be used.

The fetus is called an embryo until it shows obvious external human form. Fetal and embryonal age are thus the same and are calculated from the moment of conception or, being virtually coincidental, the moment of ovulation. Average human fetal life lasts 266 days (38 weeks) until birth.

In clinical practice, however, the duration of pregnancy is expressed as the 'gestational age', which, by convention, is calculated from the first day of the last menstrual period (LMP), i.e. the duration of amenorrhoea. Since in the usual 28-day menstrual cycle ovulation occurs on about day 14 of the cycle (day 1 being the first day of menstruation), gestational age is thus 14 days greater than fetal age and the average length of gestation until birth is 280 days (40 weeks, or about 9 calendar months and 7 days).

Fetal age is, of course, what really matters, but it is rarely feasible to define when ovulation occurred; the LMP is the only readily available reference point, hence the use of gestational age. Unfortunately, due to variation in the menstrual cycle, gestational age is often not simply equal to the duration of amenorrhoea, while other misleading factors are also common in practice. The calculation of gestational age often has to be corrected in the light of new evidence during pregnancy or even afterwards. The correction is always aimed, however, at bringing gestational age into line with fetal age (i e. the latter plus 14 days).

The Ovary

Embryology

Primordial germ cells differentiate very early in fetal life, no later than 5 weeks' gestation (i.e. 3 weeks after conception). They develop at the root of the yolk sac situated ventrally and at about 10 weeks' gestation migrate by amoebic movement, probably directed by chemotaxis, via the gut mesentery to the genital ridges situated dorsally. The germ cells become situated in the cortex of the primitive ovary (rather than in the medulla as occurs in the testis). The cortex is derived from coelomic epithelium, which also gives rise later to the granulosa cells of the ovarian follicles. The medulla is derived from mesenchyme, which later invades the cortex, thus restricting the coelomic epithelium to a thin surface layer, and gives rise to the theca cells that come to surround the follicles. The ovarian germ cells enlarge into oogonia and multiply enormously to about 7 million at 20 weeks' gestation, probably due to the very high levels of fetal gonadotrophins at this time. The oogonia undergo the first of two meiotic divisions to become primary oocytes (haploid) and remain in this stage, incapable of further multiplication, until eventually fertilized by sperm. Thus the number of oocytes can only diminish, and damaging agents have a permanent effect. The number normally falls to about 2 million at birth and 0·5 million at puberty, but a few oocytes remain even after the menopause. (In contrast, spermatogonia remain capable of mitosis throughout life.) Each oocyte becomes surrounded by a single layer of flattened coelomic epithelial (granulosa) cells, and the whole structure is called a primordial follicle.

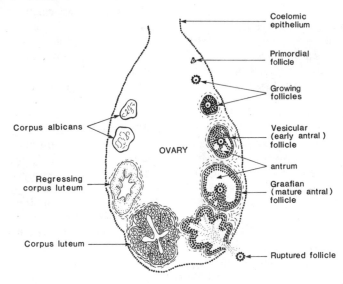

Fig. 1.1. Diagrammatic representation of the stages of ovarian follicular maturation and regression.

Follicular Growth in the Adult

This is depicted in *Fig.* 1.1. Primordial follicles grow initially by enlargement of the oocyte and the granulosa cells multiply to form a continuous membrane of cuboidal cells, eventually a few layers thick, around the oocyte. The surrounding fibrous layer of cells becomes vascularized to form the theca interna, but no blood vessels penetrate the granulosa membrane. Fluid collects in vesicular spaces (or antra) in the granulosa membrane, and the growing antra eventually coalesce into one. Further enlargement of the antral follicle is associated with the isolation of the oocyte on top of a mound (cumulus) of granulosa cells which becomes stalk-like. The oocyte becomes surrounded by a distinct layer of columnar granulosa cells (the corona radiata). The follicle, now called a Graafian follicle, is 1—1·5 cm in diameter, and has formed a swelling on the surface of the ovary, ready for rupture. Rupture occurs by enzymatic erosion, not as a pressurized explosion. The oocyte, still surrounded by its corona radiata, is thus gently released and is immediately engulfed by tubal fimbriae and transported rapidly by ciliary action into the Fallopian tube. The collapsed follicle is quickly converted into the corpus luteum by hyperplasia and swelling of the granulosa cells, the layers of which are now for the first time penetrated by blood vessels from the theca interna. The swollen granulosa cells now contain yellow pigment and so are called lutein cells. If the follicle fails to rupture it may still become partly luteinized by LH but this process can never be complete unless the follicle has been drained. If the oocyte is not fertilized the corpus luteum ceases function after 12—14 days and then slowly degenerates (so slowly that the remains of two or three such corpora lutea may be present in either ovary), ultimately becoming a fibrous structure, the corpus albicans. If fertilization and implantation occur the embryonic trophoblast secretes a gonadotrophin (human chorionic gonadotrophin, HCG) which maintains the corpus luteum.

The Control of Follicular Growth and Ovulation

A small proportion of follicles is always at the 'growing' stage. As 'growing' follicles mature further or become atretic they are replaced. The mechanism controlling this is not known, but basal amounts of gonadotrophin are required to stimulate the initial growth of the oocyte, which in turn probably stimulates the development of the surrounding granulosa membrane. Development to the antral stage is initiated by the cyclically increased secretion of FSH that occurs after puberty. Further maturation of antral follicles depends also on oestrogen (particularly oestradiol) which is secreted by the follicle itself under the influence of LH (see Fig. 1.2). About 20 antral follicles start to develop in each cycle but usually only one proceeds to maturity. The cause of the atresia in the others is unknown but may be due to capture of the blood supply within the ovary by the follicle that, by chance, advances more quickly than the rest. The blood supply is diverted by the high local concentration of oestrogen. Thus in what probably starts as an equal race (to develop) a small accidental advantage, which must inevitably occur, would rapidly be increased. Whatever the mechanism, there is no doubt that the follicle itself plays an essential part in the control of its own development. The hormones within the follicle probably mediate the final process of follicular rupture, stimulated by the LH surge, and induce the further maturation of the oocyte that is essential for fertilization to occur. It is clear that although gonadotrophins stimulate the follicles in various ways, the follicles themselves control the whole process by negative and positive feedback on gonadotrophin release.

The number of 'growing' follicles that proceed to the antral stage, and the number of antral follicles (usually one) that proceed to maturity and ovulation in any cycle, depend on the magnitude and duration of the gonadotrophin stimulus. This is normally precisely balanced, but superovulation can be induced by excessive doses of exogenous gonadotrophin.

Although the atresia of all but one antral follicle in each cycle might be explained as suggested above, the mechanism whereby no antral follicle survives in the other ovary is less clear. It is also difficult to explain why atresia of very large numbers of primordial and 'growing' follicles occurs, although it is known to be influenced by gonadotrophins, which in rats accelerate the process whereas oestrogen slows it. Why the corpus luteum, in the absence of conception, has such a remarkably constant life (13 days ± 1 (s.d.)) remains a total mystery.

Insemination, Fertilization and Implantation

The oocyte is carried along the ampullary part of the Fallopian tube by ciliary and peristaltic action. It has a life of about 24 hours but starts to deteriorate sooner, so there should ideally be sperms already available in the ampulla for fertilization.

Insemination and Sperm Transport

Sperms ejaculated near the cervix at coitus reach the tubal ampulla within 30 minutes. Although the sperms swim through cervical mucus (at about 3 mm/min), the rapid transport to the tube is probably mainly due to uterine contractions induced by oxytocin and seminal prostaglandins (orgasm is not essential). Of the many millions of sperms ejaculated only a few thousand reach the tubal ampulla. However, a steady stream is maintained, presumably by continuing uterine contractions, from a reservoir of sperms contained in cervical mucus. From the uterotubal junction the sperms are transported distally by counter currents (eddies) in the tubal fluid caused by the cilia, which all beat towards the uterus and bear the oocyte in that direction. Sperms thus reach the oocyte, not by chemical attraction but by chance. They require a few hours in the female tract to be capacitated and then deteriorate after 24 hours. They may survive, however, in an uncapacitated state in cervical mucus for some days.

Allowing for the normal life of oocyte and sperm it is obviously best that insemination occurs at intervals no longer than 2 days to achieve fertilization if the exact time of ovulation is not known. Very frequent ejaculation can reduce sperm counts critically, while continence for 10 days or more reduces sperm vitality. Thus to achieve pregnancy, coitus every 1–2 days seems to be the optimum.

Cervical mucus is an important barrier to the sperms, which only penetrate it freely during a few days just before and at ovulation. The receptiveness of the mucus is achieved by the high levels of oestrogen at this time. The oestrogen stimulates greatly increased secretion of mucus, which also becomes thinner and its mucoprotein strands become aligned in parallel, thus increasing its elasticity ('spinnbarkheit') and facilitating linear progression of sperms. It also contains salts which on drying can be seen to crystallize in typical fern-like pattern. It is important to note the presence of these features in clinical practice before drawing any conclusion when sperms in mucus examined microscopically are found to be absent or immobile. When there is little oestrogen present the mucus is scanty, viscid and cellular, and becomes so again soon after ovulation due to the antioestrogen effect of progesterone.

The high oestrogen levels that induce the changes in cervical mucus described above also stimulate increased libido in many women. However, the absent or muted cyclicity of libido in women compared with other mammals is largely due to the overriding effect of psychological factors in human sexuality. Nor are there any marked cyclical changes in the vagina or vulva that might particularly facilitate or stimulate coitus at the time of ovulation. The squamous epithelium is fully developed throughout the reproductive life of women, under the stimulus of oestrogen, and it is only the superficial cells that show cyclical change when exfoliated.

Fertilization
As soon as the sperm penetrates the oocyte fertilization by any other sperm is immediately inhibited by an unknown mechanism. Also the final meiotic division of the oocyte is completed and the second polar body is extruded. Nothing of clinical value is known about the process of fertilization, except perhaps that human sperms first need to be capacitated. When fertilization is attempted in vitro, as a means of bypassing occluded or damaged Fallopian tubes, the sperms must be capacitated by incubation for a few hours in an appropriate medium. Development of the resulting zygote beyond the blastocyst stage requires implantation into the endometrium, which remains the problematic part of the process at present.

The Zygote and Implantation
The fertilized, diploid egg is called a zygote and later, when cell differentiation commences, an embryo. The zygote is transported mainly by cilial action, which is hormone-dependent, to the uterine cavity, which it reaches after about 3 days at the morula (still solid) stage. It implants about 5 days later at the blastocyst stage. The outer cell layer (trophoblast) of the blastocyst invades the endometrium and grows rapidly as a syncytium

engulfing endometrial glands and blood vessels. The glands and blood vessels communicate with spaces which form in the syncytium and which become the future intervillous (maternal blood) spaces of the placenta. Decidual reaction in the endometrium adjacent to the trophoblast is essential if the blastocyst is to be successfully implanted. The factors that make the endometrium receptive to the blastocyst are not fully known. They clearly include, however, priming of the endometrium with large amounts of oestrogen followed for a few days by a predominance of progesterone. The oestrogen stimulus must precede fertilization; the progestogen contained in contraceptive preparations, used from the start of the cycle, interferes with endometrial development and therefore implantation. After fertilization, excessive oestrogen accelerates the passage of the zygote into the uterine cavity — by increasing tubal peristalsis — before the endometrium is receptive and can thus cause failure of implantation.

Endocrine Control of Reproduction

Ovarian Hormones

Steroids of every sort are produced by the ovary, testicle and adrenal cortex. The steroids characteristic of each of these glands predominate on account of the particular balance of enzymes present in each case. In these glands steroids are produced *de novo* from acetate via cholesterol. Active steroids are also produced in other organs from steroid precursors originating in the gonads or adrenal cortex. Thus androgen-sensitive hair follicles can produce their own androgens, and subcutaneous adipose tissue produces oestrone, which is particularly important at the start of puberty and after the menopause.

Steroids are produced in all parts of the ovary: oestrogens (especially oestradiol and oestrone) by theca cells, progesterone by granulosa cells, particularly after luteinization (i.e. in the corpus luteum) and androgens by stromal and hilar cells (hilar cells being analogous with the testicular Leydig cells). The ovary produces only small amounts of testosterone but rather more of the weak androgens, dehydroepiandrosterone (DHA) and androstenedione, than oestrogens. Progesterone is produced in relatively huge amounts.

Oestradiol is by far the most potent oestrogen. Its wide influence on reproduction has already been described, and is summarized in *Fig.* 1.2. It is essential for follicular and oocyte maturation, growth of the uterus and vagina, stimulation of cervical mucus favourable to sperms, and initial development of the endometrium in preparation for implantation. It also has some influence on libido in mid-cycle (libido in *Fig.* 1.2 being conveniently but perhaps not accurately located at the vulva!), although androgens and psychological factors generally play a bigger part. Oestrogens also contribute to breast growth (of ducts and alveoli), affect the pattern of musculoskeletal growth and subcutaneous fat distribution and exert

important controlling influences via the hypothalamus on pituitary gonadotrophin release (called 'feedback', both negative and positive). These
actions are mediated by the presence in all the target organs of specific
oestradiol-binding ('receptor') proteins within the cells. Furthermore,
oestradiol stimulates the production by the liver of a specific globulin (sex
hormone binding globulin, SHBG) to which it is strongly bound in blood
plasma, only a tiny fraction remaining free. In this way it is protected
from metabolism but available to specific receptor proteins.

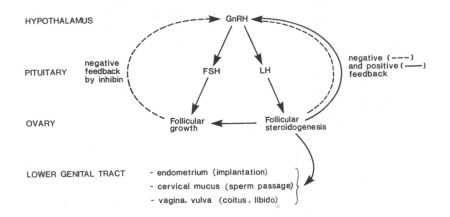

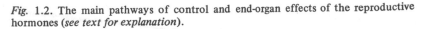

Fig. 1.2. The main pathways of control and end-organ effects of the reproductive
hormones (*see text for explanation*).

Progesterone is best known for its effect in maintaining pregnancy by
inhibiting uterine activity, but it is also essential in the final preparation of
the endometrium for implantation and it coordinates and slows the
passage of the zygote along the Fallopian tube. It has certain antioestrogen
effects, notably on endometrial proliferation and cervical mucus. Like
oestradiol (but less strongly) it exerts negative feedback, via the hypothalamus, on pituitary gonadotrophin release; it can also exert positive
feedback but only after experimental priming with oestrogen. In the breast
it stimulates alveolar growth in combination with other essential hormones.

Inhibin: the ovarian follicle produces an unidentified, non-steroidal
hormone like testicular inhibin that plays a part in the negative feedback
control of FSH release. Thus premenopausal cycles are commonly infertile
and associated with high FSH levels, despite normal steroid levels. Also, in
an uncommon condition called the 'resistant ovary syndrome' there are
absent menstrual cycles, high gonadotrophin levels, despite adequate
oestrogen levels, and bizarre abnormality of the follicles.

The Ovarian Endocrine Cycle

The ovarian endocrine cycle is of course closely related to the ovarian follicular cycle which passes through 'follicular' and 'luteal' phases. Oestradiol and progesterone levels in peripheral blood reflect secretion rate by the follicle. As shown in *Fig.* 1.3 oestradiol (and to a lesser extent oestrone) levels increase exponentially, during the antral phase of the follicles, but this only takes about 1 week before ovulation. There is no appreciable oestradiol rise in the pre-antral 'growing' phase of the follicles,

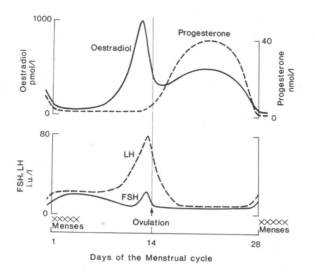

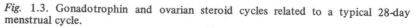

Fig. 1.3. Gonadotrophin and ovarian steroid cycles related to a typical 28-day menstrual cycle.

which starts (by an unknown mechanism) even before the previous corpus luteum ceases function. The pre-antral phase of the cycle is the most variable in duration. Oestradiol reaches a peak, only to fall sharply a couple of days before ovulation. It then increases again due to secretion by the corpus luteum to reach a lower, flatter, secondary peak, before finally falling as the corpus luteum ceases to function (unless pregnancy occurs). The average levels of oestradiol are twice as high in the luteal than in the follicular phase. Progesterone levels are low throughout the follicular phase but start to rise under the stimulus of the LH surge shortly before ovulation, increasing steadily due to secretion by the corpus luteum to reach a wide peak, and falling again in a symmetrical pattern as the corpus luteum fails.

It is not practically feasible to observe the actual occurrence of ovulation, but the steroid levels in blood provide an accurate guide. Luteal progesterone is the best index (*see* Chapter 11). Although a defective corpus luteum or a luteinized unruptured follicle invariably reflects impairment in the preceding 'follicular' phase, it is ordinarily too difficult to 'catch' the relatively sharp oestradiol peak.

Genital Changes Dependent on Ovarian Hormones

The changes in the superficial cells of the vaginal epithelium, only recognized microscopically, and the more obvious changes in cervical mucus have already been mentioned. The most obvious event is the *menstrual cycle,* i.e. the cyclical shedding with bleeding of secretory endometrium when oestrogen and progesterone levels fall as the corpus luteum fails. The normal *endometrial cycle* consists of proliferative and secretory phases that correspond with the follicular and luteal phases of the ovarian cycle. The physical changes in the endometrium and the process of menstruation will be described in detail later.

Non-reproductive Metabolic Effect of Ovarian Hormones

Oestrogens affect nearly all other endocrine systems. By increasing their specific binding globulins in plasma, oestrogens cause an increase in the total circulating amounts of cortisol, thyroxine and progesterone, and also of iron and copper. Oestrogens also stimulate the secretion of cortisol and growth hormone, thus reducing carbohydrate tolerance despite enhancing the insulin response. Prolactin secretion is also stimulated, although without any obviously important consequence. Oestrogens and progesterone have complex but generally opposing effects on fluid and electrolyte balance, oestrogens usually causing salt and water retention. Aldosterone secretion increases in the luteal phase, perhaps to counteract the salt-losing effect of progesterone despite the presence of large amounts of oestrogen. Renin is stimulated by oestrogen and plasma triglycerides rise. Biliary secretion and excretion tend to be reduced and blood coagulability increased. The widely varied effects mentioned, nearly all due to oestrogens, are small. Some have caused varying degrees of concern, however, in relation to the long-term use of oral contraceptive preparations and postmenopausal hormone replacement, in so far as such treatment might cause or aggravate diabetes, hypertension, coronary occlusion and thromboembolism.

Gonadotrophins

The two gonadotrophins, follicle stimulating hormone (FSH) and luteinizing hormone (LH), are glycoproteins, very similar in structure to thyroid stimulating hormone (TSH) and human chorionic gonadotrophin (HCG). FSH and LH are produced by the anterior pituitary under the stimulus of gonadotrophin releasing hormone (GnRH) from the hypothalamus. FSH and LH are also stored in the anterior pituitary and can be released suddenly in large amount by a big dose of GnRH. Although gonadotrophins inhibit the secretion of GnRH by negative feedback on the hypothalamus, the main control of gonadotrophin secretion is by oestradiol and progesterone. Acting on the hypothalamus they both usually exercise negative feedback, but when the oestradiol level increases to high levels it exercises positive feedback, i.e. it induces a discharge of GnRH which leads to a release of gonadotrophins, especially LH. (Progesterone will also do this in experimental conditions but only after priming with oestrogen.) Although there appears to be only one form of GnRH, differential responses of FSH and LH occur according to the steroid environment of the pituitary.

Gonadotrophin Cycles Through Life

FSH and LH are detectable in blood throughout life, levels being elevated in four distinct cycles:

1. In the fetus during the first half of pregnancy very high levels of gonadotrophins are present and probably stimulate the huge proliferation of oogonia. The levels fall to low as the fetal hypothalamus appears to become sensitive to negative feedback by placental oestradiol.
2. Soon after birth, with the removal of placental oestradiol, gonadotrophin levels rise, but the ovaries are now resistant to them (although not completely). Gonadotrophin levels fall slowly again over about 4 years, perhaps due to increasing hypothalamic sensitivity to negative feedback.
3. They rise gradually again from about 8 years of age, possibly due to a reverse trend in the sensitivity of the hypothalamus to negative feedback, but the mechanism is not known. A gradual rise in oestradiol from the stimulated ovarian follicles follows. Cyclical fluctuation of oestradiol and FSH then develops, the one being a mirror of the other owing to negative feedback, and menstruation may occur. Finally hypothalamic sensitivity develops to positive feedback by rising high levels of oestradiol and the LH surge characteristic of the adult cycle occurs resulting in ovulation (see below).
4. At the menopause, depletion of ovarian primordial follicles results in deficiency of oestradiol (and probably inhibin) leading to very high gonadotrophin levels.

The Adult Gonadotrophin Cycle

The adult gonadotrophin cycle is shown in Fig. 1.3. As steroid levels in blood fall at the end of the luteal phase the FSH level rises due to release of negative feedback on the hypothalamus. LH rises less, the release of LH being more sensitive to negative feedback. With the secretion of oestradiol by antral follicles the FSH level falls again gradually. Although this fall occurs just when follicular maturation is accelerating, it seems that the follicle is more sensitive to FSH because of the presence of oestradiol, which may also help to capture the available FSH for the most advanced follicle by increasing the local blood flow (see above).

As oestradiol levels in blood increase so the LH level rises slightly due to increasing positive feedback, and finally there is a huge surge lasting about 24 hours. This is accompanied by a smaller surge of FSH, caused by the same discharge of GnRH, although it does not seem to have any function. The LH surge stimulates the final maturation of the Graafian follicle and rupture about 24 hours later and induces luteinization of the follicle.

Because of the high levels of both oestradiol and progesterone the LH and FSH levels fall sharply to lower levels in the luteal than in the follicular phase.

In clinical practice FSH and LH can be readily assayed and their measurement is essential in distinguishing the causes of amenorrhoea (see Chapter 10). Human gonadotrophin extracted from the urine of postmenopausal women can be used to induce follicular maturation in certain anovulatory states (see Chapter 10).

Gonadotrophin Releasing Hormone

Gonadotrophin releasing hormone (GnRH) is also called FSH- and LH-releasing hormone and often abbreviated as FSH/LH-RH, LHRH or LRH. It is a simple decapeptide, secreted by the hypothalamus and transported via the hypophyseal portal blood vessels to stimulate production and release of FSH and LH by the anterior pituitary. The control of GnRH secretion is mainly by oestradiol and progesterone, and to a lesser extent FSH and LH, by feedback mechanisms already described.

The assay of GnRH is difficult. In clinical practice the distinction between hypothalamic and pituitary failure, which occur rarely, can only be made by the difference in gonadotrophin response to injected synthetic GnRH. Whether synthetic GnRH has a useful therapeutic place in the induction of ovulation has yet to be determined.

Prolactin

Prolactin is a polypeptide in the form of a single long chain, resembling growth hormone and human placental lactogen. There appear to be a few analogous forms in the human, which may account for some of the difficulties in its radioimmunoassay. It is secreted by the anterior pituitary and its control is discussed more fully in Chapter 10. There is no significant variation in prolactin levels in blood through the menstrual cycle. Although prolactin seems to be essential for normal follicular steroidogenesis, particularly in the corpus luteum, very low levels in blood do not interfere with ovulation. Hyperprolactinaemia, however, inhibits ovarian function, both directly and by interfering with gonadotrophin secretion, and is a common cause of ovulatory failure. The recognition of the existence of human prolactin, its measurement by radioimmunoassay and the ability to treat hyperprolactinaemia represent one of the most exciting recent advances in medicine.

Melatonin
Melatonin and related substances are secreted by the pineal body which is inhibited by light. Melatonin somehow acts via the brain to inhibit gonadal function and to influence various light-dependent cycles. It may thus play a part in the timing of puberty. Destruction of the pineal body, for instance by a tumour, can cause precocious puberty.

The Endometrium and Menstruation

The Endometrium and Endometrial Cycle

The normal endometrial cycle (*see Fig.* 1.4) consists of proliferative and secretory phases that correspond with the follicular and luteal phases of the ovarian cycle. Under the influence of oestrogen alone the endometrial glands and stroma both proliferate, mitoses being commonly seen on histology, the glands becoming longer as the endometrium thickens. The endometrial spiral arterioles (not shown in *Fig.* 1.4) become increasingly

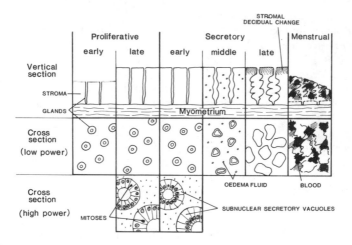

Fig. 1.4. Histological changes in the endometrium through the menstrual cycle (*see text for description*).

coiled, developing out of proportion to the needs of the endometrium but adapted to the future needs of expected trophoblast. Progesterone then blocks endometrial proliferation and induces secretory changes, indicated initially by secretory vacuoles building up below the nuclei of the glandular epithelium. Later the secretion pushes past the nuclei into the glandular lumen, distending the glands, and the stroma becomes loose and oedematous. Finally the glands become grossly distended and tortuous, and near the endometrial surface the stromal cells become enlarged, pale and close-packed, rather like the much more marked decidual change that occurs when a blastocyst implants. The spiral arterioles are now at their peak development. In the absence of fertilization the fall in luteal steroid levels causes spasm of the spiral arterioles and necrosis and shedding of the endometrium (except for the basal layer, from which regeneration occurs under the influence of oestrogen in a new cycle). Between the dense basal layer of endometrium, which is relatively inactive, and the dense superficial layer due to stromal decidual change, the middle layer of distended glands appears to be spongy. It is particularly marked in pregnancy, and is called the 'decidua spongiosa'.

Menstruation

Menstruation is the shedding of secretory endometrium with bleeding which occurs at the end of each ovarian cycle if conception has not taken place. The shedding of non-secretory endometrium associated with ano-vulatory cycles or withdrawal of exogenous steroids like the contraceptive 'pill' is not true menstruation, but this cannot be distinguished in practice.

Shortly before menstruation the endometrium (except its basal layer) shrinks and becomes disrupted due to the reduction in its ovarian endocrine support. At the same time the endometrial spiral arterioles undergo spasm leading to blanching of the endometrium, but this may be the result rather than the cause of the endometrial disruption, caused by the local release perhaps of catecholamines. The arteriolar spasm is then relaxed inter-mittently, leading to the main bleeding that occurs with menstruation. Thus the arterioles control the amount of bleeding, but as yet there is no effective therapeutic control of them. The total blood lost at each men-strual period is on average 40 ml, the normal range being 20–60 ml.

The menses thus consist mainly of blood and also the fragmented endometrium including its secretions and tissue exudate. The menses are characteristically fluid, the blood unclotted. This is probably due to fibrinolysins released by the damaged tissue, which dissolve the initial clot. When clotting occurs it is usually because of excessive bleeding, presumably due to relative lack of local fibrinolysins. A rough guide to the amount of blood lost is the number of towels or tampons needed to contain it: normally no more than 12 are needed for the whole period.

The menstrual period lasts on average 4 days, the normal range being 2–6 days. The menstrual loss occurs with a distinct pattern during this time, starting suddenly and increasing to peak flow on usually the second day, then diminishing gradually to a watery loss as the endometrium regenerates.

The menstrual cycle, measured from the start of one menstrual period to the next, lasts on average 28 days, diminishing gradually from 30 days at 20 years of age to 27 days at 40 years. The distribution of cycle length around the mean is skewed, the normal range being 21–42 days. It should be noted that this variation occurs not only between individuals but also within any individual, even amongst those women who consider themselves to be 'as regular as clockwork'. The variation is much greater, with a particular tendency to long cycles, in the first 5 years after the menarche and the last 8 years before the menopause. The shortest possible fertile cycle, i.e. associated with ovulation, is 21 days, because it takes at least 7 days for follicular ripening and the luteal phase consistently lasts about 14 days.

The onset of menstruation is the easiest point of reference in practice, and the day menstruation starts is called day 1 of the cycle. In an average 28-day cycle ovulation thus occurs on day 14 (*see Fig.* 1.3).

Further Reading

Amelar R. D., Dubin L. and Walsh P. C. (1977) *Male Infertility*. Philadelphia, Saunders.

Austin C. R. and Short R. V. (ed.) (1972) *Reproduction in Mammals. No. 1: Germ Cells and Fertilization; No. 3: Hormones in Reproduction*. Cambridge, Cambridge University Press.

Mishell D. R. and Davajan V. (1979) *Reproductive Endocrinology, Infertility and Contraception*. Philadelphia, F. A. Davis.

Short R. V. (ed.) (1979) Reproduction. *Br. Med. Bull.* 35(2), 97–204.

Yen S. S. C. and Jaffe R. B. (1978) *Reproductive Endocrinology*. Philadelphia, Saunders.

Chapter two

Reproductive Anatomy

GYNAECOLOGICAL ANATOMY
Genital Embryology

Fig. 2.1 shows the stage of development of the urogenital tract at 10 weeks' gestation prior to sexual differentiation. The development of testes

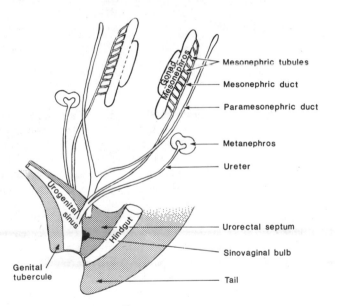

Fig. 2.1. Combined sagittal and oblique views of urogenital system at 10 weeks' gestation, just before sexual differention.

results in regression of the paramesonephric (Müllerian) ducts due to the local effect of a substance as yet unidentified (an experimentally transplanted testis inhibits the paramesonephric duct only on the side on which it is implanted). The mesonephric (Wolffian) duct develops into the epidydimis and vas deferens. The development of ovaries, however, leads to differentiation of the paramesonephric ducts into the uterine (Fallopian) tubes on each side, and of the uterus by fusion of the ducts in the midline. The embryology of the ovary has already been described in detail in Chapter 1.

Incomplete fusion of the paramesonephric ducts results in a variety of uterine anomalies as shown in *Fig.* 2.2. These may interfere with placentation, leading to abortion, and in late pregnancy often cause abnormal fetal lie, leading to difficulties in labour.

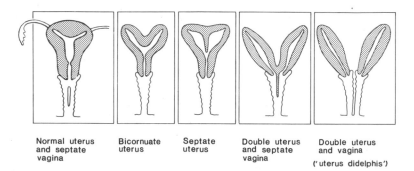

| Normal uterus and septate vagina | Bicornuate uterus | Septate uterus | Double uterus and septate vagina | Double uterus and vagina ('uterus didelphis') |

Fig. 2.2. Common anomalies of the uterus and vagina due to varied degrees of nonfusion of the embryonic structures from which they originate.

At 10 weeks' gestation the fused portion of the paramesonephric ducts has already invaded the urorectal septum, where it later meets the upgrowths of the paired sinovaginal bulbs from the urogenital sinus (which is endodermal in origin) and these form most if not all of the vagina. These bulbs are solid, and failure of cavitation can lead to various degrees of vaginal atresia, while non fusion of the bulbs results in a vaginal septum or double vagina (*Fig.* 2.2).

In the absence of testes the mesonephric ducts regress, but their remnants occasionally form cysts. These occur, as would be expected, closely adjacent to the Fallopian tubes and to the anterolateral border of the uterus and upper vagina where they are called cysts of Gärtner's duct. The remains of the mesonephric tubules, close to the ovaries, are called the 'epoophoron' and give rise to parovarian cysts.

The metanephric duct (ureter and renal pelvis) develops by budding out from the lower end of the mesonephric duct and later becomes separately inserted into the upper part of the urogenital sinus as it expands to form the trigone of the urinary bladder.

The sexual differentiation of the external genitalia depends on testosterone. Thus in the male the genital tubercle (*see Fig.* 2.1) grows into the phallus, and the genital swelling and folds on each side (not shown in *Fig.* 2.1) fuse to form, respectively, the scrotum and the floor of the penile

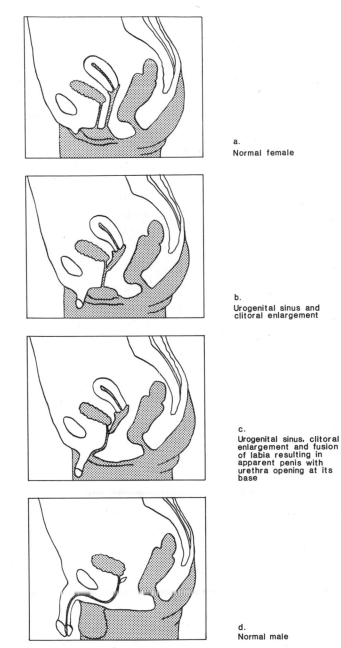

a.
Normal female

b.
Urogenital sinus and
clitoral enlargement

c.
Urogenital sinus, clitoral
enlargement and fusion
of labia resulting in
apparent penis with
urethra opening at its
base

d.
Normal male

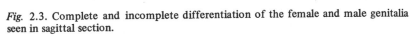

Fig. 2.3. Complete and incomplete differentiation of the female and male genitalia
seen in sagittal section.

urethra (*Fig.* 2.3*d*). Absence of testosterone results in failure of phallic growth, and non fusion of the genital swelling and folds resulting in the open vestibule of the vulva (*Fig.* 2.3*a*) and separate labia. Differentiation of the external genitalia is complete and unalterable by 16 weeks' gestation. Before this time, however, inadequate testosterone in the male, or excessive androgen in the female (e.g. exogenous or due to adrenal cortical hyperplasia), may result in intermediate stages of development called intersex, as for example in *Figs.* 2.3*b* and 2.3*c* (*see* Chapter 9). The appearances at birth in such cases may be difficult to interpret or, worse, wrongly interpreted.

Associated Anomalies

As expected from the embryological relationships, developmental anomalies of the genital tract are often associated with anomalies of the urinary tract, such as aberrant or double ureter and pelvic kidney, and occasionally of the anus, which may open into the perineum or vagina.

The Vulva

The vulva is the name for the female external genitalia and is depicted in *Fig.* 2.4. It is bordered by the mons veneris anteriorly and the labio-crural folds posterolaterally. The vaginal introitus is usually closed due to apposition of the labia majora but may gape to some degree in parous women. The labia minora are hairless and virtually simple folds of skin, but they contain highly vascular tissue which may become turgid when sexually excited. The labia minora fuse anteriorly to form the prepuce of the clitoris, which is thus usually hidden. The clitoris consists of erectile tissue analogous with the penis and also becomes turgid (to a varying degree) when sexually excited (*see* Chapter 7). The vestibular bulbs, analogous with the corpus spongiosum in the male, extend backwards from the clitoris deep to the bulbocavernosus muscle (*Fig.* 2.5).

The depression between the labia minora, into which open the urethra and vagina, is called the vestibule. The ducts of Bartholin's glands also open onto it posterolaterally (*Fig.* 2.5). The anterior limit of the vestibule is the clitoral prepuce and the posterior limit is the fourchette (*Fig.* 2.4). The latter is a skin-fold at the posterior aspect of the vaginal introitus. To allow delivery of a baby the fourchette has to stretch very greatly, and the perineum has to stretch both laterally and anteroposteriorly, the anus being pushed backwards.

1. *Innervation* of the vulva is illustrated in *Fig.* 2.5.
2. *Arterial supply* is mainly by the internal pudendal artery (from the internal iliac artery) which accompanies the pudendal nerve from the ischial spine, and anteriorly by the superficial external pudendal artery (from the femoral artery).
3. *Venous drainage* accompanies the arteries.

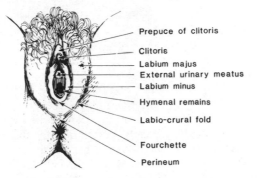

Prepuce of clitoris

Clitoris

Labium majus

External urinary meatus

Labium minus

Hymenal remains

Labio-crural fold

Fourchette

Perineum

Fig. 2.4. The vulva.

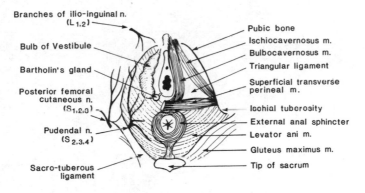

Branches of ilio-inguinal n.
$(L_{1,2})$

Bulb of Vestibule

Bartholin's gland

Posterior femoral
cutaneous n.
$(S_{1,2,3})$

Pudendal n.
$(S_{2,3,4})$

Sacro-tuberous
ligament

Pubic bone

Ischiocavernosus m.

Bulbocavernosus m.

Triangular ligament

Superficial transverse
perineal m.

Ischial tuberosity

External anal sphincter

Levator ani m.

Gluteus maximus m.

Tip of sacrum

Fig. 2.5. Structures lying deep to the vulva.

4. *Lymphatic drainage* accompanies the blood vessels and is mainly to the superficial inguinal nodes, thence to the deep inguinal and external iliac nodes; from deeper structures lymphatics accompany the pudendal vessels to the internal iliac nodes. There is free cross-drainage between the two sides, but due to the distinct embryological origin of the vulva the lymphatic field is sharply demarcated peripherally by the labio-crural folds (*Fig.* 2.4).

The Pelvic Floor

The pelvic floor consists of all tissues from (and including) the pelvic peritoneum to the vulva and perineum, but in terms of support the most important structures are the levator ani muscles and the pelvic fascia.

The Muscles

The perineal group of muscles (*Fig.* 2.5) are minor structures of little importance in the woman. They share common insertion with some fibres of the anal sphincter, and in particular with the levator ani muscles, into a midline raphe called the perineal body (*Fig.* 2.6*a*). This is a fibromuscular structure which has to stretch very greatly with the perineum to allow delivery of a baby (*Fig.* 2.6*b*), and is then frequently torn or deliberately incised (episiotomy, *see* Chapter 14).

The levator ani muscles (*Fig.* 2.5) form a sling from the lateral pelvic walls, the fibres passing downwards and posteriorly to their insertion in the perineal body, coccyx and sacrum. They form a floor for the pelvis which slopes downwards, medially and forwards, this shape having an important influence on the way the fetal head is channelled in the process of delivery. The levator ani muscles pull the perineal body upwards and forwards thus acting as a sphincter and support for the vagina, which is consequently normally held in a slight S-shape (*Fig.* 2.6*a*); by supporting

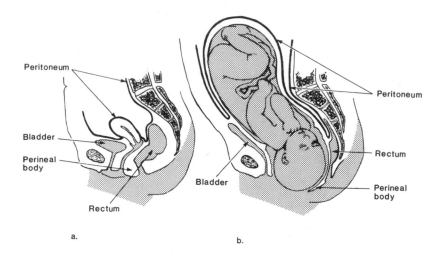

Fig. 2.6. Sagittal view of the genital tract in (*a*) non-pregnant stage, and (*b*) pregnancy, as the fetal head is distending the vagina and perineum just before delivery.

the vagina they also support and raise the bladder neck and can be used to prevent micturition. The levator ani muscles are voluntary but are reflexly relaxed during micturition and defaecation and are reflexly contracted when otherwise straining, such as when coughing. Their innervation is from S2, 3, 4 via the pudendal nerve (*Fig.* 2.5).

Below and lateral to the levator ani muscle on each side, and between it and the lateral pelvic wall, is the ischiorectal fossa filled with fatty connective tissue. Above and medially is the pelvic fascia, with the urethra, vagina and anal canal passing downwards between the muscles in the midline.

The Pelvic Fascia and Ligaments

The pelvic fascia is the connective tissue lying between and above the levator ani muscles and below the pelvic peritoneum. It envelops on each side the vagina and cervix (where it is called the parametrium) and the bladder neck in front. It is condensed radially to form distinct supports for the pelvic organs. The most important are the transverse cervical or cardinal ligaments, but there are also the pubocervical ligaments that pass antero-posteriorly on each side of the bladder neck and the uterosacral ligaments that pass from the uterine isthmus (between cervix and uterine body) backwards around the sides of the rectum.

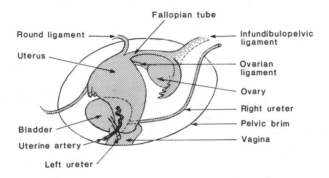

Fallopian tube

Round ligament — Infundibulopelvic ligament

Uterus — Ovarian ligament

Ovary

Right ureter

Pelvic brim

Bladder — Vagina

Uterine artery —

Left ureter

Fig. 2.7. The pelvic organs viewed obliquely through the pelvic brim from above, left and behind.

The pelvic fascia extends thinly and loosely upwards between the peritoneal folds of the broad ligament running laterally from each side of the uterus. This ligament is wrongly named because it has no supportive function, being merely peritoneum draped over the round ligament, Fallopian tubes and ovarian ligaments which pass laterally from the uterine horns (*Fig.* 2.7). The infundibulopelvic ligaments (*Fig.* 2.7) are, similarly, non-supportive continuations of the broad ligaments to the pelvic brim posterolaterally, carrying the ovarian blood vessels. Within the pelvic fascia pass all the branches of the internal iliac arteries with the veins and lymphatics to or from the pelvic organs (e.g. the uterine artery, *Fig.* 2.7).

The Ovarian Ligaments and Round Ligaments

These are conveniently described here (*Fig.* 2.7) but are not part of the pelvic fascia. The two, being continuous via the uterine horn, are analogous with the gubernaculum testis. Thus the round ligaments curve forwards to the internal inguinal ring and thence pass to the labia majora. The ovarian ligaments suspend the ovaries. The round ligaments have little supportive function but tend to keep the uterine body pulled forwards in its usual anteverted attitude.

The Ureters

The ureters (*Fig.* 2.7), after entering the true pelvis beneath the infundi-bulopelvic ligament on each side, pass vertically down the pelvic side wall to the ischial spine and turn forwards and medially in the pelvic fascia beneath the uterine artery in the base of the broad ligament to reach the bladder. They pass close by the sides of the cervix, just above the lateral vaginal fornices, where they are crossed by the uterine arteries. The ureters are prone to damage when dividing the uterine arteries at hyster-ectomy, by irradiation of or invasion by cervical carcinoma, by operations on densely adherent inflammatory swellings near the base of the broad ligaments, and when dividing the ovarian vessels in the infundibulopelvic ligaments.

The Pelvic Organs

The Vagina

This is an elastic, fibromuscular tube lined by non-keratinized squamous epithelium that passes upwards and backwards from the introitus at the vulva. It is about 10 cm long, variably distensible, and is normally closed by apposition of its anterior and posterior walls. It is held in a slight S-shape (*Fig.* 2.6*a*) by the tone of the levator ani muscles acting through the perineal body, which can be used voluntarily (and involuntarily, sometimes out of fear) to close the vagina forcibly. The cervix protrudes into its upper anterior wall, dividing the vaginal vault into anterior, posterior and lateral fornices.

Its anterior wall is related to the urethra and bladder neck, to which it is connected by dense connective tissue, and to the cervix. Posteriorly it is related to the perineal body and rectum. Its vault is directly adjacent to the deepest part of the uterorectal peritoneal pouch (pouch of Douglas), through which pelvic structures can be palpated (*Fig.* 2.6*a*), and to the ureters and uterine blood vessels on each side (*Fig.* 2.7). Laterally the vagina is separated from the levator ani muscles by pelvic fascia in which run the vaginal branches of the uterine arteries and accompanying venous plexuses.

The squamous epithelium has no special structures, unlike skin, but exudation through it keeps the vagina moist. The degree of exudate depends on the vascularity of the vaginal wall, which is determined by oestrogen. The normal vaginal contents appear creamy, being a mixture of tissue exudate, exfoliated cells and cervical mucus. Full maturation of the epithelium depends on oestrogen, while the addition of progesterone induces minor superficial cytological changes. Under the influence of oestrogen the mature (superficial) cells contain glycogen which is metab-olized to lactic acid by lactobacilli, which are normal commensals in the vagina. Thus the vagina is normally acidic (pH 4–5) in women of reproductive age, especially in pregnancy. However, there is a pH gradient due to the alkaline cervical mucus, and during menstruation the vagina is almost neutral.

The Uterus

The uterus consists of a body and a cervix. The body is pear-shaped and flattened anteroposteriorly giving its cavity a flat, triangular shape. It connects with the Fallopian tube at each horn (cornu) and the domed top of the uterine body, between its horns, is called the fundus. The cervix is a canal about 2·5 cm long, being narrowest at its internal os where it joins the uterine body. This junctional region is called the isthmus although not anatomically distinct. The length of the uterine cavity including the cervix is about 6 cm in nulliparous women and up to 8 cm in parous women. The walls of the uterus are 1–1·5 cm thick and consist almost entirely of smooth muscle, the myometrium. The muscle fibres are arranged into three layers: inner and outer longitudinal fibres inserted into cervical connective tissue, and a much thicker middle circular layer. There are relatively few muscle fibres in the lower part of the cervix, which consists more of fibrous connective tissue. Thus it is the internal os that determines the competence of the cervix as a sphincter in pregnancy.

The endometrium is the mucosal lining of the uterine body and consists of tubular glands set in a highly cellular stroma. Under the influence of oestrogen and progesterone it undergoes distinct cyclical changes as described in Chapter 1, consequently varying in thickness from 1 to 5 mm.

The endocervix is the mucosal lining of the cervix. It is thrown into an arborescent pattern of folds, or crypts, and consists of a columnar surface epithelium and underlying loose cellular stroma, which is also very vascular, giving the endocervical mucosa a bright red colour. Its appearance remains constant through the ovarian cycle, but the amount and properties of its mucus secretion show distinct changes (see Chapter 1).

The ectocervix is the stratified squamous epithelium covering that part of the cervix projecting into the vagina and is continuous with the vaginal epithelium in the fornices. It is smooth and, being relatively thick, looks opaque and dull pink, in contrast to the bright, velvety endocervical mucosa with which it is continuous near the external cervical os. The line of demarcation between ecto- and endocervix is called the squamo-columnar junction. It is in this area that cervical epithelial dysplasia and carcinoma usually start and from which diagnostic cytology smears should therefore be taken. This junction often occurs far outside the external cervical os, and in pregnancy endocervical mucosa may cover much of the vaginal portion of the cervix. This appears to be the result of differential growth of the underlying cervical parenchyma, mediated by oestrogen. The junction may return to the external os (and even within it after the menopause), partly by involution of the underlying tissue but mainly by squamous change (metaplasia) in the mucosa due to physical exposure in the vagina.

The uterus is covered by closely adherent peritoneum (*Fig.* 2.6*a*) all over its posterior surface, including the supravaginal portion of the cervix, and over the anterior surface of the body. Anteriorly the peritoneum is reflected off the isthmus onto the bladder and laterally is reflected off the sides of the uterus in a vertical line to form the two layers of the broad ligaments.

The uterus is related anatomically over its peritoneal surface to intestinal loops and omentum. Anteriorly its isthmus is attached to the bladder by loose connective tissue which at Caesarean section is easily divided to afford approach to the lower part ('lower segment') of the uterus. Laterally (*Fig.* 2.7) it is related to its appendages (or adnexa) contained within the broad ligaments (Fallopian tubes and ovaries, round and ovarian ligaments) and to the parametrium below and the structures passing through that tissue (ureters and uterine blood vessels).

The main uterine supports are the transverse cervical ligaments (*see* Pelvic Fascia *above*). The round ligaments tend to hold the uterus forwards (in 'anteversion') but are elastic.

The Fallopian Tubes (Oviducts)
These are two, thin, muscular tubes connecting the uterine cavity via each uterine horn with the peritoneal cavity (*Fig.* 2.7). Each is about 10 cm long and consists of four parts: the intramural part (2 cm) traversing the uterine wall, the narrow isthmus (3 cm), the wider ampulla (5 cm) and the infundibulum (fimbriated opening). Each tube is contained within the upper border of the broad ligament, but the infundibulum and part of the ampulla are free and tend to curve around the ovary. The lumen of the tube is very narrow in the isthmus and intramural parts; in the ampulla it appears to widen but is filled by intricate folds of the mucosal lining (endosalpinx). The endosalpinx is a delicate columnar epithelium consisting of secretory and ciliated cells that help to support and propel both egg and sperms (*see* Chapter 1).

The Fallopian tubes are related over their peritoneal surface to the ovaries and loops of intestine. At their inferior margin within the broad ligaments they are related to an arcade of anastomosing utero-ovarian blood vessels and to remnants of the mesonephric ducts (e.g. epoophoron) which sometimes develop cysts that can stretch the tubes greatly.

The Ovaries
Their structure and function have been described in Chapter 1. They are flattened ovoids 3–4 cm long suspended from the back of the broad ligament by a wide mesovarium that carries the ovarian blood vessels, lymphatics and nerves, and from the uterine horn by the narrow ovarian ligament (*Fig.* 2.7).

Blood Supply

The uterine artery is a branch of the internal iliac artery and passes medially in the pelvic fascia, crossing above the ureter to reach the uterine isthmus (*Fig.* 2.7). Vaginal and cervical branches pass downwards, and the main uterine trunk passes tortuously up the side of the uterus to anastomose with the ovarian artery in the broad ligament.

The ovarian artery is a branch of the aorta on each side and enters the pelvis in the infundibulopelvic ligament (*Fig.* 2.7) from which it passes into the broad ligament beneath the Fallopian tube. It supplies the ovaries and tubes and finally anastomoses with the uterine arteries.

The internal pudendal artery is the terminal branch of the posterior division of the internal iliac artery. Passing out of the pelvis through the greater sciatic foramen it curves around the ischial spine and proceeds forward in the ischiorectal fossa to supply the vulva, which is also supplied anteriorly by the superficial and deep external pudendal arteries, branches of the femoral artery (*see* The Vulva *above*).

Correspondingly named veins accompany the arteries but are usually multiple or as plexuses, notably the pampiniform plexus in the broad ligament which drains into the ovarian and uterine plexuses.

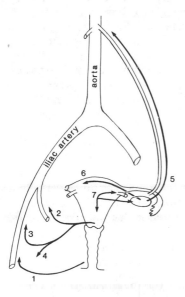

Fig. 2.8. The main lymphatic pathways draining the genital tract, numbered as described in the text.

Lymphatic Drainage

The main pathways, accompanying the major arteries, are outlined in *Fig.* 2.8. The lower vagina drains, like the vulva (*see above*), into the inguinal nodes (shown as pathway 1). The cervix drains via lymphatics in the pelvic fascia (parametrium) to the internal iliac nodes (2) and to the external iliac nodes (3) including the obturator node (4). The ovaries drain along the course of the ovarian vessels (5) to the para-aortic nodes and also across the midline via the uterine fundus (6). The uterine body drains (7) as for both the ovaries and cervix and also via the round ligaments to the super-ficial inguinal nodes. Early metastasis of endometrial and ovarian carcinoma to relatively distant lymph nodes is one reason why lymphatic block excision or radiotherapy is usually unsuitable treatment for these con-ditions, unlike cervical carcinoma (*see* Chapter 6).

Innervation
The nerve supply of the vulva has been described above (*see Fig.* 2.5).

The uterine body and cervix are fairly insensitive except to distension, which causes not only severe pain but can also cause reflex vasovagal shock that is occasionally fatal. The nerve supply is entirely autonomic, both sympathetic (via the presacral plexus) and parasympathetic (via the pelvic plexus), the cervix being innervated more than the uterine body. There are both sensory and motor nerves. Pain from the uterine body is referred to the lower abdomen and from the cervix to the sacral area. The myometrial response to catecholamines depends on the presence of both α-receptors (excitatory, mainly stimulated by noradrenalin) and β-receptors (inhibitory, by adrenalin). The balance of effect depends on hormones: oestrogens enhance α-adrenergic effect, and progesterone β-adrenergic. Some 'β-mimetic' drugs can be used to inhibit labour when it occurs prematurely.

The ovaries and Fallopian tubes are supplied by sympathetic and parasympathetic nerves accompanying the ovarian blood vessels from the pre-aortic plexus. The ovaries are sensitive only to compression, as on bimanual palpation, but the tubes are sensitive to all the usual stimuli.

The Urinary Bladder and Urethra
These structures are important in gynaecology because urinary disorders including incontinence are commonly associated with genital disease, and they can be damaged at operations on the genital organs.

The bladder is a hollow muscular organ lined by transitional epithelium with an inverted pyramidal shape when empty. When full it is domed and has a capacity of at least 500 ml. The ureters enter the trigone of the bladder obliquely, thus affording valve-like protection against reflux of urine while being able to fill the bladder by peristaltic action.

The urethra is a muscular tube 3—4 cm long lined by transitional epithelium, except in its lower part where the epithelium is squamous and, like the vulva, is affected by oestrogen. The paraurethral glands open onto the posterior wall of the urethra and are commonly the site of chronic infection.

There are three coats of smooth muscle in the bladder wall. The inner longitudinal fibres run into the urethra as the detrusor muscle, which thus opens up the bladder neck and upper urethra at the onset of micturition.

The middle layer is circular and does not extend to the urethra. The outer layer is longitudinal and continues spirally around the urethra, thus helping to maintain urethral resistance. The maintenance of urinary continence, however, especially on straining as when coughing, is not fully understood. It probably occurs by a valve effect rather than by a sphincter, the urethral pressure being raised simultaneously with intravesical pressure by transmission of intra-abdominal pressure. The valve effect is further aided by the reflex contraction of voluntary muscles: the levator ani muscles, which, acting through the perineal body, compress the urethra and bladder neck and accentuate the posterior urethrovesical angle (*Fig.* 2.6*a*), and the external urethral sphincter.

Micturition is mainly controlled by a parasympathetic nervous reflex via S3, 4 which after infancy becomes conditioned at cerebrocortical level. Thus afferent impulses generated by bladder distension and weight on the trigone are normally inhibited unconsciously and, in response to rising stimulation, consciously. The reflex can also be inhibited by painful stimuli, thus explaining the urinary retention which occurs so commonly after vaginal surgery or after perineal laceration at childbirth.

The mechanism of micturition involves: (1) reduction of cortical inhibition, (2) voluntary relaxation of the pelvic floor, leading to lowering of the bladder neck and straightening of the posterior urethrovesical angle, (3) detrusor contraction, leading to urine entering the upper urethra and causing (4) reflex contraction of the bladder, (5) voluntary contraction of the pelvic floor and external urethral sphincter to squeeze the urethra 'dry' again and finally (6) reapplication of cortical inhibition. Urinary incontinence is thus commonly caused by (1) loss of the posterior urethrovesical angle, associated with vaginal prolapse, (2) loss of urethral resistance, associated with aging, and (3) detrusor irritability due to infection or psychological factors (*see* Chapter 4).

The Rectum and Anus

These structures are only important because their proximity to the genital tract exposes them to the risk of associated damage (*see Fig.* 2.6). The anal sphincter and canal can be lacerated during childbirth; the rectum can be damaged when repairing prolapse of the posterior vaginal wall; and pelvic suppuration tracks down to the pouch of Douglas resulting in adhesions between uterus and the upper rectum which can endanger the upper rectum at hysterectomy.

Orientation of the Pelvic Organs

The key to the orientation of the pelvic organs within the pelvis is the position of the cervix, which is situated in the very centre of the bony cavity of the true pelvis (*see Fig.* 2.6*a*), firmly suspended by the strong transverse cervical ligaments. The uterus can pivot about this point; it is usually angled forwards at 90° to the vagina ('anteverted') as shown in

Fig. 2.6*a*, but filling of the bladder rotates it backwards, while in some normal woman the uterus may be usually thus 'retroverted'. The body of the uterus may also be angled (flexed) on the cervix; thus it is usually 'anteflexed' (*Fig.* 2.6*a*) as well as anteverted, and when retroverted is often also 'retroflexed' (being then palpable in the pouch of Douglas and often painful on sexual intercourse). The position of the ovaries and Fallopian tubes depends of course on that of the uterus.

In pregnancy the uterine body rises into the abdomen, but the cervix remains supported in the centre of the pelvic cavity and the fetal head cannot descend until the cervix is dilated. When the head remains at a higher level, however, it cannot be due to the cervix but may be due to obstruction at the pelvic brim.

The key to the orientation of the pelvic organs with respect to the rest of the body is the angle of inclination of the pelvic brim. This is 55–60° from the horizontal in a standing woman as shown in *Fig.* 2.6 (but steeper in a Negress). Thus the uterus is normally situated above the symphysis

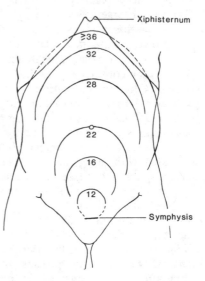

Fig. 2.9. The usual height of the uterine fundus in the abdomen at different stages (weeks) of gestation.

pubis; it is not palpable in the lower abdomen because it is far back. In early pregnancy the uterus grows forwards in the axis of the pelvic brim to come within reach at 10–12 weeks' gestation. At this stage the uterus lies horizontally upon the empty bladder, but can be displaced upwards to misleadingly high levels when the bladder is full. The bladder should therefore be emptied before any attempt to assess uterine size. After 14 weeks' gestation the uterus grows vertically in the abdomen (*Fig.* 2.9). In late pregnancy the fetal head passes backwards to enter the pelvis in the axis of the pelvic brim (*see Fig.* 2.13). It does not move vertically downwards (i.e. towards the mother's feet) until it is just about to be delivered (as in *Fig.* 2.6*b*).

OBSTETRICAL ANATOMY
The Uterus

In pregnancy the uterine body is distended by the gestation sac to a globular shape until 14 weeks' gestation, becoming elongated thereafter. With the cervix supported at its fixed level (*see* Orientation *above*), the fundus of the growing uterus moves forwards until it reaches the anterior abdominal wall where it can be first palpated at 10–12 weeks. After 12–14 weeks it moves vertically upwards within the abdomen as shown in *Fig.* 2.9. At 16 weeks the fundus has reached half-way from symphysis pubis to umbilicus, at 22 weeks to the umbilicus and at 28 weeks half-way to the xiphisternum. After 32 weeks it expands mainly outwards. Thus assessment of gestational age by palpation of the urerus is best done by bimanual pelvic examination up to 14 weeks, by the fundal height until about 32 weeks and thereafter by the feel of the size of the fetus itself; after 36 weeks it is not possible to distinguish further.

The enlargement of the uterus stretches the round ligaments and ovarian attachments vertically, carrying the ovaries into the flanks. Because of disproportionate distension of the uterine fundus the round ligaments only reach half-way up the uterus at the end of pregnancy ('term').

During pregnancy the uterus enlarges twentyfold in mass and its length reaches 30 cm at term. The myometrium grows mainly by hypertrophy of the individual fibres, which increase tenfold in length; the total mass increases from about 50 g to 1000 g but the thickness of the myometrium does not increase. The endometrium undergoes marked secretory change, becoming spongy (Chapter 1), and is called the decidua. The uterine isthmus expands with the uterine body to accommodate the pregnancy sac but remains below the sac and has to be dilated with the cervix in labour. The isthmus and cervix together constitute 'the lower segment' of the uterus. The cervix becomes very vascular (hence its typical blue appearance) and oedematous. In the intercellular ground substance there is a vast increase in suspended water (i.e. as droplets) which loosens the collagen fibres and permits them to slide so as to enable the remarkable dilation that the cervix undergoes in labour. All the pelvic organs undergo marked increase in vascularity and the venous plexuses become greatly distended.

The Bony Pelvis

It is only the true pelvis (i.e. the part below the pelvic brim, or inlet) that is obstetrically important, being the rigid part of the birth canal. As shown in *Fig.* 2.13, from the inlet (A) to the outlet (C) its axis curves through about 50°. Also, its cross-sectional shape changes; *Fig.* 2.10 shows that the normal ('gynaecoid') brim is slightly wider in its transverse diameter than its anteroposterior (A-P) diameter (the 'obstetric' conjugate), whereas the outlet is wider in the A-P than the transverse. Note that the coccyx, whatever its angle, does not restrict the outlet because it is flexible. The mid-pelvis (level B, *Fig.* 2.13) is round in cross-section. The outlet may be restricted by the ischial spines in some cases. Normally, however, although the interspinous diameter is narrower than the others the spines are behind the centre of the outlet; although they appear prominent from above (*Fig.* 2.10a), viewed from below they are hidden by the sacrotuberous ligaments (*Fig.* 2.10b).

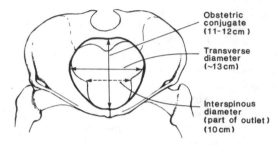

a. Pelvic brim viewed perpendicularly to its axis from above

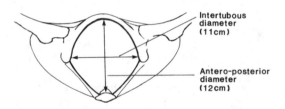

b. Pelvic outlet viewed from below

Fig. 2.10. Views demonstrating the main pelvic diameters.

The cross-sectional shape of the pelvis largely determines the position of the fetal head at each level (*see* Chapter 14 on Mechanism of Delivery). The inlet is the most restricting part of the pelvis because the outlet can be expanded in all directions by movement at the sacroiliac joints and symphysis pubis. Thus if the fetal head will pass through ('engage' in) the pelvic brim it will certainly pass through the outlet of a normally shaped pelvis. The lower normal limit of the obstetric conjugate is 10 cm. In general, if the sacral promontory cannot be reached on vaginal examination the obstetric conjugate must be greater than 10 cm. The actual diameter being measured digitally is from the lower border of the symphysis pubis to the sacral promontory and is known as the diagonal conjugate.

Abnormalities of pelvic shape are an uncommon problem now in this country thanks to relatively good nutrition. In any case there is no place now for the difficult labour and delivery that would have to be conducted to overcome the gross abnormalities commonly associated with rickets which were seen in the past. The most common abnormality now experienced is straightness, or even convexity, of the anterior surface of the sacrum in its upper part instead of its normal marked concavity. In such a pelvis the shortest A-P diameter of the pelvic inlet (the obstetric conjugate) may lie below the pelvic brim. Previous fracture is an occasional cause of pelvic distortion.

The Fetus

The widest part of the fetus is across the shoulders, but these can be angled through the mother's pelvis and rarely cause obstruction. Thus the

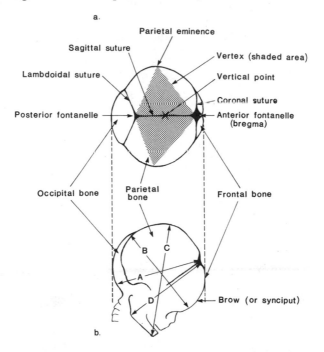

Fig. 2.11. Anatomical features of the fetal head looking (*a*) onto the vertex and (*b*) from the side. The particular diameters A, B, C, D are described in the text.

biggest part in effect is the fetal head. It is fortunate that it usually presents first.

The fetal head is not quite spherical, and since some of its diameters in the sagittal plane (*Fig.* 2.11*b*) are greater than its maximal transverse diameter (*Fig.* 2.11*a*), the degree of flexion or extension of the head at the neck determines the ease (or difficulty) with which the head can negotiate the mother's pelvis. The important anatomical features are shown in *Fig.* 2.11, which portrays the head almost fully flexed, the chin nearly on the chest; if the head as in *Fig.* 2.11*b* is turned upside down and then viewed from below, as it would appear from the vagina, it would be seen as in *Fig.* 2.11*a*. When the head presents with different degrees of flexion or extension the features to be found on vaginal examination are shown in *Fig.* 2.12.

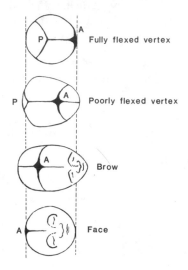

Fig. 2.12. The features of the fetal head presenting vaginally with different attitudes of the head. The fontanelles are marked A (anterior) and P (posterior).

The particular sagittal diameter (*Fig.* 2.11*b*) that must negotiate the pelvis associated with each type of presentation (*Fig.* 2.12) is:

Fig. 2.12	*Fig.* 2.11*b*	
Fully flexed vertex	A Suboccipitobregmatic	9·5 cm
Poorly flexed vertex	B Occipitofrontal	11·5 cm
Brow	C Mentovertical	13·5 cm
Face	D Submentobregmatic	9·5 cm

Thus the most favourable presentations of the head to negotiate the pelvis are when fully flexed or fully extended. The presenting shape is then almost exactly round, since the maximal transverse diameter (between the parietal eminences – biparietal diameter) also measures about 9·5 cm at term.

The brow at term presents such a large diameter that it is undeliverable vaginally. It is therefore very important to recognize a brow presentation as soon as possible. Unfortunately the diagnosis is difficult on abdominal palpation and is also commonly missed in labour until it is advanced. This is because at early dilatation of the cervix it may not be possible to identify more than the anterior fontanelle (recognized by its four radiating sutures), which is mistakenly assumed to indicate a poorly flexed vertex (compare with the brow in *Fig.* 2.12). Never diagnose a vertex presentation until the posterior fontanelle (which is triradiate) has been identified on vaginal examination.

Cephalopelvic Relationships

Position

When the fetal head presents as usual by the vertex, its relationship to the maternal pelvis is defined by the orientation of the sagittal suture and the occiput, which can be palpated vaginally. The head, as indicated by the sagittal suture, may occupy (1) the transverse, (2) the anteroposterior or (3) an oblique diameter of the pelvis.

The exact position of the fetal head is defined by the orientation of the occiput, which is recognized on vaginal examination by the posterior fontanelle (*see Figs.* 2.11 and 2.12). Thus in each of the pelvic diameters just described the head may be in the (1) left or right occipitolateral position, (2) occipito-anterior or occipitoposterior, (3) left occipito-anterior or right occipitoposterior, or right occipito-anterior or left occipitoposterior, respectively. The commonest position in which the head enters the pelvis is occipitolateral (curiously, more commonly with the occiput on the left rather than the right); the commonest position at delivery is occipito-anterior.

When the face presents, the positions are described in a similar manner but orientated to the chin; thus mento-anterior, etc. The positions of a brow presentation are not described in any particular way.

Level

Since the brim is usually the narrowest part of the pelvis the ability of the fetal head to negotiate it is of prime importance. When the greatest diameter of the head has passed through the brim it is said to be engaged. Since in general the head can be assumed to be symmetrical it is engaged when at least half through the brim. On abdominal palpation, the level of the head is best described in terms of the proportion (conventionally in fifths) remaining above the pelvic brim (*Fig.* 2.13). Thus when the head is just engaged there is only between 2/5 and 3/5 above the brim, but 5/5 when wholly above.

When examining the abdomen with the patient lying on her back (as in *Fig.* 2.13), the uppermost point of the head (arrowed in the figure) is in the same horizontal plane as the anterior border of the symphysis pubis when the head is engaged, assuming the usual angle of inclination of the pelvic brim. When the head is 5/5 above the pelvic brim the upper point of the head is 5 cm above this horizontal, the head at term being about 10 cm in diameter. This (arrowed) point is thus an accurate guide to the level of the head in relation to the pelvic brim. It is of course situated over the

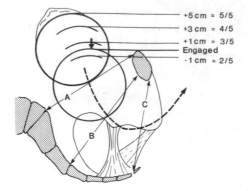

Fig. 2.13. Combined sagittal and internal views of the pelvis with the mother lying on her back. The anteroposterior diameters are shown of the pelvic inlet (A, 'obstetric conjugate'), mid-cavity (B) and outlet (C), and the axis of the pelvis throughout (dotted line). The fetal head is shown as a sphere in the sagittal plane of the mother, the face being usually to one side. The relation of the level of the head to the pelvic brim (expressed as fifths of the head remaining above the brim) can be accurately derived in practice by relating the uppermost point of the head (arrowed) to the horizontal plane of the anterior (palpable) point of the symphysis pubis (*see text*).

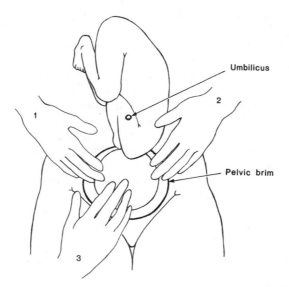

Fig 2.14. The surface markings on the maternal abdomen of the pelvic brim and fetus in particular the fetal head, and the points to seek on palpation as described in the text.

centre of the pelvic brim and can be palpated by backward pressure with the right hand half-way between symphysis pubis and umbilicus as shown by position 3 in *Fig.* 2.14. Inaccuracy in assessing the level of the head in relation to the pelvic brim occurs (1) with the occipitoposterior position, in which the face projects forwards in the midline, and (2) in a Negress, in whom the steep inclination of the brim projects the whole head forwards.

In practice, before assessing the level of the head it is necessary first to confirm the presentation, and this is done more easily with the two hands in positions 1 and 2 as in *Fig.* 2.14. A rough idea of the depth of the head in the pelvis can also be obtained in this way.

The level of the head can be related clinically to the ischial spines on vaginal examination. The ischial spines being on either side, it is necessary to imagine a line joining them to which the lowermost part of the head can be related. As *Fig.* 2.13 shows, the head is about 2 cm above the spines when just engaged in the brim. This assumes, however, that there is no moulding of the head; when this occurs, as in prolonged labour associated with cephalopelvic disproportion (the head too large for the pelvis), the head may be elongated to well below the spines yet remain unengaged. Thus the level of the head must never be assessed vaginally without assessing it abdominally also.

Further Reading
Austin C. R. and Short R. V. (ed.) (1972) *Reproduction in Mammals. No. 2: Embryonic and Fetal Development.* Cambridge, Cambridge University Press.
Myerscough P. R. (1976) *Munro Kerr's Operative Obstetrics,* 9th ed. London, Baillière and Tindall.

Chapter three

Gynaecological Inflammatory Disorders and Pelvic Pain

Inflammatory disorders of the genital tract may result in sterility, menstrual disorders, chronic pelvic pain, deep dyspareunia and general ill health. Prompt diagnosis and treatment of acute inflammations are important in minimizing the' risk of long-term problems. Dyspareunia is the term given to painful intercourse and dysmenorrhoea the term for painful periods.

The Vulva

The vulva is remarkably resistant to bacterial infection. It is constantly contaminated by urine and vaginal secretions and by faecal organisms from the rectum. Faulty hygiene is also common. Inflammation of the vulva (vulvitis) may occur alone or in conjunction with inflammation of the vagina (vulvovaginitis).

Vulvitis

Clinical features are of severe irritation (pruritus vulvae) with intense burning pain, exacerbated during micturition. On examination the labia may be tense and swollen, and there may be accompanying vaginal discharge. The introitus is often so tender that vaginal examination and coitus are impossible. Causes of vulvitis are mechanical trauma, chemical agents, infections and skin diseases.

Vulvitis is almost always aggravated by mechanical trauma from scratching in response to pruritus, although not itself a primary cause. The liberal use of chemical agents such as antiseptics (commonly Dettol) in the bathwater, vaginal deodorants or biological washing powders may cause chemical or allergic reactions; various medicaments used to treat or alleviate the vulvitis may themselves cause adverse reactions and further aggravate the vulvitis. Nylon underwear which fails to absorb moisture, particularly if worn in association with tights and trousers, adds to maceration of vulval skin predisposing to vulvitis. Poor hygiene may be a contributory factor, for example in elderly obese women who are unable to carry out personal toilet adequately after defaecation.

Vulval Infections
Candida albicans (monilia or 'thrush') may case acute vulvitis alone but more commonly presents as vulvovaginitis. However, it is not infrequently found at routine examination without symptoms. Candidiasis of the vulva causes irritation and burning but in the vagina produces a thick white cheesy discharge (*see below*). Exacerbation of the infection is found in association with pregnancy, diabetes mellitus, the use of oral contraceptives and antibiotic therapy. Treatment is with antifungal vaginal pessaries for 2 weeks (e.g. nystatin or miconazole). Antifungal cream is useful to soothe the acutely inflamed vulva allowing the pessary to be inserted. Recurrence is frequent and may occur from the gastrointestinal tract which acts as a reservoir, or following intercourse, since candida may be harboured asymptomatically under the prepuce. Systemic antifungal therapy and cream for use on the penis by the patient's consort are necessary. The avoidance of tight clothing and nylon underwear, especially in the summer, alleviates the condition since candida thrives in a warm, moist, poorly ventilated area. The modern fashion for prolonged wearing of a swimsuit which is kept moist by its wearer swimming from time to time is commonly associated with candidal infection, especially in the tropics.

Trichomoniasis of the vagina (*see below*) causes a profuse frothy vaginal discharge which causes a secondary vulvitis and severe pruritus. Treatment is with oral metronidazole 200 mg t.d.s. for 7 days for the patient and her consort.

Since the organism is transmitted sexually and harboured asymptomatically reinfection may occur if the partner is not treated. Alcohol should be avoided during treatment since metronidazole has an Antabuse (disulfiram BP)-like action. Metronidazole can be given safely in pregnancy but, as with most drugs, should be avoided in the first trimester.

Threadworm infestation usually occurs in children. The worms migrate from the anus at night causing severe irritation. The trauma of scratching produces lesions which are readily infected. Treatment is with piperazine sulphate.

Lice (pediculosis pubis) are transmitted by intimate bodily contact and cause irritation in the pubic hair region. Treatment is with DDT powder.

Herpesvirus hominis type 2 (herpes genitalis) infection of the vulva is sexually transmitted. The primary lesion is a group of small vesicles with surrounding erythema and oedema, producing an intense localized vulvitis and commonly vaginitis and cervicitis too. Idoxuridine may counter the infection in the earliest stage, but the diagnosis is not usually made till later when there is no effective treatment. Herpesvirus type 2 may be implicated in the genesis of cervical dysplasia and carcinoma (*see* Chapter 6).

Condylomata accuminata (or venereal warts) are papillary warty growths of the vulva, vagina, perineum and occasionally cervix. These lesions are caused by a virus and have a narrow base (unlike the broad-based condylomata lata of syphilis — *see below*). They produce a profuse irritant discharge and often coexist with *trichomonas vaginalis*. Treatment is with topical podophyllin 10 per cent in tincture of benzoin for smaller lesions. It is important to protect the surrounding skin with Vaseline before painting with podophyllin. Since podophyllin is absorbed and is teratogenetic it should not be used in pregnancy. Cautery, cryosurgery or excision may be needed for larger lesions.

Bacterial Infection of the Vulva
Infection of the hair follicles of the vulva (folliculitis) is common and especially in diabetic patients may become chronic. It is treated with antibiotics in the early stages, but if an abscess forms it requires incision. Sebaceous cysts are common and if secondarily infected may lead to abscess formation.

Skin Diseases
The vulval skin may be involved as part of generalized skin disease such as psoriasis or eczema or may be affected alone. In the obese, intertrigo often affects the vulva because of the moisture of the labial and inguinal regions. Specific localized vulval skin diseases (the vulval dystrophies — *see* Chapter 6) present as abnormal-looking skin in association with pruritus. Clinical diagnosis is difficult and any abnormal vulval skin should be biopsied to determine the nature of the lesion and exclude malignant change.

Pruritus vulvae is a common symptom for which often no cause is found. The identifiable causes are listed:

> Urinary
> > incontinence
> > glycosuria
> > pyuria
> Vulvovaginal
> > discharge
> > chemicals   ⎫ direct or allergic
> > mechanical ⎭
> Anal
> > haemorrhoids
> > threadworms
> Skin disease
> > generalized
> > localized
> Systemic disease
> > uraemia
> > hepatitis
> > Hodgkin's disease
> Psychosomatic
> > sexual frustration

Identifiable causes should be sought and treated specifically. If no cause is found, palliative treatment is necessary and may help in cases where the cause is known. The avoidance of hot baths and clammy nightwear is advised; the wearing of gloves at night may reduce the trauma caused by scratching, and cotton underwear, stockings and skirts are to be preferred to tights and trousers. In non-infected cases 1 per cent of hydrocortisone cream is effective but should be used in short (7–14 day) courses.

A *Bartholin's cyst* is a dilatation of the duct of Bartholin's gland. It is usually unilateral, and asymptomatic unless infected. Treatment is by excision or marsupialization (eversion of the cyst wall and suturing it to the overlying skin), since infection and formation of a Bartholin's abscess are common. The gland itself is rarely involved in the inflammatory process, but if infected the dilated duct is excruciatingly tender. Staphylococci, streptococci and *E.coli* are the common organisms involved. Treatment is by incision of the abscess and marsupialization in the acute phase, excision being impossible due to inflammation. The gonococcus may infect the duct and the gland bilaterally but acute Bartholinitis rarely presents in this way clinically. Recurrent infection in the older woman should raise the rare possibility of carcinoma of the gland (*see* Chapter 6).

The Vagina

Vaginitis may occur if the protective physiological environment of the vagina is altered. To maintain its normal bacterial flora the vagina has to be moist and acid. The glycogen produced in the squamous epithelial cells of the vagina in response to oestrogen is broken down to lactic acid by Döderlein's bacilli (lactobacilli). The pH of the adult vagina is normally about 4. This acidity provides protection against invasion by other micro-organisms such as staphylococci and streptococci. The acidity and thickness of the squamous epithelium of the vagina are optimal during reproductive life, but can be impaired in some circumstances. Increased secretion of cervical mucus, which is alkaline, will raise the vaginal pH allowing pathogenic bacteria to grow. Vaginal douches and deodorants may also disturb vaginal pH. Antibiotics disturb the normal vaginal flora and Döderlein's bacilli are particularly sensitive to broad-spectrum antibiotics. Vaginal acidity is reduced during menstruation and in the immediate puerperium. Before puberty and after the menopause low oestrogen states result in a vaginal epithelium with low glycogen content.

Vaginitis

The symptoms are vaginal (often vulvovaginal) itching or soreness, superficial dyspareunia and most commonly discharge. The nature of the discharge varies with the cause of the vaginitis, usually in a characteristic way.

Causes of vaginitis and vaginal discharge:
Infective
   Trichomonas
   Candida albicans
   bacterial
Atrophic
   postmenopausal
   pre-pubertal
Mechanical
   foreign body
Chemical
   douches, pessaries
Excretions
   urinary and faecal fistulae

Additional causes of vaginal discharge:
Secretions
   excessive cervical mucus
   semen
Inflammation
   cervicitis
Neoplasms
   carcinoma of the cervix or vagina
   necrotic polypfibroid, or cervical

Infective Vaginitis
Trichomonas vaginalis: The typical discharge of trichomonal infection is watery greenish yellow and foamy with an unpleasant, characteristic smell. It is usually associated with constant vulvovaginal irritation. The diagnosis is made by taking a drop of the discharge, placing it in normal saline and examining it under the microscope. The pear-shaped protozoan with its undulatory membrane and long flagellum will then be seen (*Fig.* 3.1). Treatment is described on page 37.

An appreciable number of women with trichomonal vaginitis will also have gonorrhoea, and steps should be taken to exclude this by taking swabs and slides from urethra, cervical canal and vaginal vault for appropriate culture and Gram staining.

Fungal infection: This is usually with *Candida albicans* (monilia or 'thrush') and frequently involves the vulva also. The discharge is thick, white and cheesy. It is not offensive but is intensely pruritic and also causes soreness and dyspareunia. Treatment is as for candidal vulvitis on page 37.

Bacterial vaginitis: A wide range of bacteria can be isolated from the normal vagina and it is relatively rare for the symptoms of vaginitis to be closely related to bacterial infection, and to be cured by appropriate antibiotic therapy. Bacterial vaginitis is usually associated with trauma in young women or with foreign bodies in young girls and old women. Culture of the discharge yields a mixed bacterial flora, and the causative organism may be missed unless special culture media are used, e.g. *Haemophilis vaginalis* requires a medium containing blood and even so is only

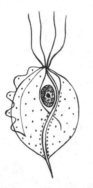

Fig. 3.1. Trichomonas vaginalis.

grown with difficulty. As a result the diagnosis is often not defined, but if associated with a foreign body the condition resolves on its removal.

Atrophic Vaginitis
In the postmenopausal woman the vaginal skin is thin, the pH alkaline and the protective lactobacilli are lacking. Irritation, soreness and dyspareunia are common symptoms. Discharge is not a prominent feature but bleeding may be. If the postmenopausal woman complains of bleeding, whether just spotting or frank blood, a full examination including a diagnostic curettage is mandatory, even if atrophic vaginitis is present. Endometrial carcinoma must be excluded before starting treatment for atrophic vaginitis with systemic or local oestrogen. Local oestrogen is absorbed anyway. Pessaries or jelly containing lactic acid may also be helpful.

Vaginitis Due to Foreign Body
In children the foreign body may be a small object inserted deliberately or fluff or toilet tissue which accumulates due to poor hygiene and forms a nidus about which debris collects. During reproductive years it is usually a forgotten tampon, although the literature contains many amusing reports of items that have been removed from the vagina, ranging from champagne corks and wine glasses to bicycle pumps and milk bottles. In the postmenopausal woman it is commonly a forgotten ring pessary. In all cases a profuse offensive discharge is produced.

Chemical Vaginitis
Direct or allergic reactions may occur in the vagina to chemicals contained in douches, deodorants, bath salts, medications and biological washing

powders as well as to latex condoms. Vaginal soreness is the predominant symptom, discharge being less of a feature. On examination the vagina looks red and inflamed. Careful questioning is necessary to discover the cause.

Excretions Causing Vaginitis
Contamination of the vagina with urine from a vesicovaginal fistula or faeces from a rectovaginal fistula causes a secondary vulvovaginitis. The treatment is to deal with the underlying cause, but barrier creams and antiseptic vaginal douches may help.

Inflammation of the cervix (cervicitis) causes a discharge and often secondary vulvovaginitis.

Neoplasms causing vaginitis: serosanguinous discharge may arise from carcinoma of the vagina, the cervix, endometrium and even rarely, the Fallopian tubes.

Secretions Causing 'Discharge'
Excessive cervical secretion may occur in psychosomatic conditions such as the pelvic congestion syndrome or due to excessive cervical ectopy (*see below*). The 'discharge' will not cause soreness, irritation or be blood stained. Frequently the patient complains of its offensive odour. This is often not detected by anyone else. The 'discharge' produces a mixed growth of normal bacterial vaginal flora when cultured. It is not uncommon for women, early in their coital experience, to complain of a 'discharge' after intercourse. It has none of the characteristics of a pathological discharge, only the characteristic smell of semen. Explanation regarding the volume and liquefaction of semen together with reassurance that 'not all the sperm have run away' is usually all that is required.

The Cervix

Acute Cervicitis
Acute inflammation of the cervix is rare and is usually gonococcal or herpetic in origin and usually asymptomatic.

Chronic Cervicitis
Chronic inflammation of the cervix is a more common cause of symptoms. It is often associated with pelvic pain, discharge and dyspareunia. On examination the cervix is enlarged by multiple Nabothian follicles (*see* Chapter 6) and these retention cysts have become secondarily infected, usually with a mixed bacterial flora. Of the rarer specific causes of chronic cervicitis chlamydia is the most common but is only detectable if special culture techniques (viral) are used. Tuberculosis is a rare cause.

Management
A cervical smear should be sent for cytological examination and cervical

and vaginal swabs sent for bacteriological culture because, rarely, antibiotic therapy may be indicated for a specific organism.

The cervix should be cauterized. This may be done with cryosurgery or electrocautery in the out-patient clinic, but more extensive lesions requiring deeper diathermy cautery or conization need to be treated under general anaesthesia. Cautery will cause a marked discharge for 7—10 days and may be associated with secondary haemorrhage around the tenth day as the slough is shed. Rarely cervical stenosis results from cautery.

The Uterus

Infection of the cervix is common, but spread of infection to the uterus is inhibited by the cervical mucus. The upper part of the cervical canal and the endometrial cavity are usually sterile. The endometrium is remarkably resistant to infection, and while salpingitis is common, endometritis is rare. Infection virtually only occurs when the endometrium is damaged following abortion or parturition. After the menopause secretions may collect in the endometrial cavity if the internal os is stenosed and occluded by atrophy, carcinoma or radiation. This collection becomes infected and is called a pyometra. The symptoms are commonly a purulent or serosanguineous discharge and sometimes abdominal pain and fever. On examination the uterus is enlarged and may be tender, softened and cystic. Treatment is dilatation of the cervical canal to drain the uterus and diagnostic curettage to exclude an underlying carcinoma.

Pelvic Inflammatory Disease (PID)

This broad term covers infection involving the tubes, ovaries and parametrium. Other intrapelvic organs, particularly gut, may also be involved, usually as a result of adhesions. Pelvic inflammatory disease may be acute or chronic.

Causes of PID

1. *Ascending* infection through the genital tract, usually related to coital activity (e.g. *Neisseria gonorrhoeae*) but may be due to chlamydia, and other organisms.
2. *Direct* infection due to trauma, usually related to abortion or delivery. Infection is due to gut or vaginal commensals, quite commonly with anaerobic organisms (e.g. bacteriodes).
3. *Blood-borne infection,* classically tuberculosis, usually at the time of puberty, which produces a silent chronic salpingitis, but theoretically any bacteraemia may result in pelvic foci of infection.
4. *Transperitoneal infection* from, for example, appendicitis or diverticulitis.

Acute Pelvic Inflammatory Disease

In salpingitis the Fallopian tubes are congested and oedematous and on microscopy are found to be infiltrated by polymorphonuclear leucocytes. A seropurulent exudate collects in the tubal lumen resulting in fibrinous adhesions, obliteration of the lumen and blockage of the tube. Pus escapes from the abdominal ostium initially, but when this becomes blocked the tubes distend and typically become retort shaped. This collection of pus in the tube is known as pyosalpinx. The leakage of pus into the peritoneal cavity may produce an acute pelvic peritonitis. Spread of the infection to the ovary is called salpingo-oophoritis and may result in the formation of a tubo-ovarian abscess. A collection of pus in the pouch of Douglas is called a pelvic abscess.

CLINICAL FEATURES OF ACUTE PID

Symptoms: The patient complains of lower abdominal pain and fever. The pain is typically bilateral. She may also have a vaginal discharge and admit to deep dyspareunia.

Examination: Abdominal examination in the acute phase characteristically reveals rebound tenderness over the pelvis and both iliac fossae. On vaginal examination there is bilateral adnexal tenderness, but the tubes are not initially palpable because they are soft and only slightly swollen. Moving the cervix produces pain (excitation pain). The differential diagnosis is from other causes of acute abdominal pains such as appendicitis, ectopic pregnancy and twisted ovarian cysts. In all these instances the features are usually unilateral: salpingitis in a woman with both tubes is never so, except in rare cases of tuberculosis.

In the next stage of the pathological process of pelvic inflammatory disease the diagnosis is more apparent since pyosalpinges and a tubo-ovarian abscess are palpated as bilateral tense, tender, relatively immobile masses. It is imperative that examination at this stage is carried out with utmost gentleness to prevent rupture of the masses leading to generalized peritonitis. If acute salpingitis is treated fairly early in its pathological process after blockage of the fimbrial end of the Fallopian tube, then the tube may fill with clear fluid of tubal secretions forming a hydrosalpinx as opposed to the smaller thick-walled, pus-filled tube of the pyosalpinx. Fluid from the hydrosalpinx is sterile on culture.

Diagnosis: This is made definitively by laparoscopy, which affords the opportunity to take swabs from the fimbrial ends of the tubes and from the pouch of Douglas. The swabs must be transported urgently to the laboratory in the appropriate media for aerobic and anaerobic culture, and a slide sent for Gram staining. Swabs from the lower genital tract are often unhelpful but should nevertheless be cultured, particularly for *Neisseria gonorrhoeae.* For that reason swabs should be taken not only from the vagina but also from the cervical canal and urethra.

TREATMENT OF ACUTE PID
Acute salpingitis is treated with high doses of antibiotics, bed rest and analgesia. Treatment should be started without waiting for bacteriological confirmation of the causative organism. Early diagnosis and treatment is vital to preserve function of the Fallopian tubes. Once an exudate starts to form, the fimbriae become oedematous, lose their cilia, fuse and may eventually block the ostium. Even if the ostium is patent, subsequent fertility is grossly jeopardized.

Chronic Pelvic Inflammatory Disease
If treatment of the acute stage is delayed or is inadequate then fibrous adhesions between tube, ovary and surrounding structures usually follow, including fixed retroversion of the uterus. The mucosal folds and cilia of the tubes are destroyed.

CLINICAL FEATURES OF CHRONIC PID
Chronic salpingitis or inactive adhesions involving other pelvic organs are associated with persistent lower abdominal pain which is usually bilateral. The patient may also complain of persistent vaginal discharge, menorrhagia and deep dyspareunia. On examination a low grade fever may be found. There is generalized lower abdominal tenderness which is usually worse on one side, but rebound tenderness is absent. On pelvic examination unilateral or bilateral firm tender adnexal masses are palpable. The masses are often adherent to the uterus and the pelvic side wall. Acute exacerbations are common and should initially be treated conservatively (i.e. with antibiotics, analgesics and rest) but may eventually require surgical intervention. Pelvic clearance (total hysterectomy and bilateral salpingo-oophorectomy) is the treatment of choice if the patient is prepared to accept loss of her fertility. It may be possible to conserve one or both ovaries in some cases. Operations to restore fertility, restoring tubal patency and tubo-ovarian anatomy, have little success. Such operations must be done in the quiescent phase of the disease.

Parametritis (Pelvic Cellulitis)
Inflammation of the parametrium occurs as a result of trauma to the cervix during delivery or abortion, or after injury to the vagina or cone biopsy of the cervix. Parametritis may develop by spread from an infected tube and ovary (salpingo-oophoritis) or from an infected uterus (endometritis). Clinically the patient complains of constant deep unilateral pelvic pain. She is pyrexial. On abdominal examination there is unilateral tenderness low down in one or other iliac fossa. On vaginal or, preferably, rectovaginal examination a thickened tender mass can be palpated extending from the uterus to the pelvic side wall. This interferes with the mobility of the uterus. Treatment is with high doses of antibiotics and anti-inflammatory agents. The condition can be bilateral.

Venereal Diseases

The study of venereal disease is concerned with infective and inflammatory lesions which are sexually transmitted. Some of these infections are endemic in almost every part of the world. Syphilis, on the other hand, has become sporadic in certain countries, but there is a tendency for epidemics of venereal disease to arise in any country during times of strife.

Venereal disease must be seen in its social setting related to society and its customs, as well as to individuals' attitudes and behaviour. Particular epidemiological problems occur in connection with the infectious carrier, sexual promiscuity, perversion, prostitution, homosexuality and in relation to the law. In the UK the law recognizes three infections as venereal: gonorrhoea, syphilis and non-specific urethritis.

Chancroid, granuloma inguinale and lymphogranuloma venereum are transmitted venereally in a large proportion of cases. They are usually described together since they are causes of genital 'sores'; they are relatively rare and they tend to be limited to warmer climates and sea-board cities. Here we will consider gonorrhoea and syphilis as they have an important bearing on normal gynaecological and obstetrical practice. The student is referred to a textbook of venereology for the rarer sexually transmitted diseases which may present gynaecologically.

Gonorrhoea

During the years 1946—55, mainly as a result of the availability of antibiotics, the incidence of gonorrhoea and syphilis fell progressively and dramatically in nearly all countries. It was thought at that time to be a dying disease. Since then, however, there has been a steady increase and the World Health Organisation has now declared gonorrhoea to be out of control. Apart from the common cold it is the most prevalent infectious disease.

The increase in gonorrhoea has occurred in females rather than males, and in adolescents rather than adults. Indeed a quarter of all female cases now occur in women less than 20 years of age. The explanations for this continuing rise in incidence are:

1. Development of drug-resistant gonococci.
2. A shift in populations.
3. Increased promiscuity among the young.

The last is the most important and is creating serious medicosocial problems.

The causative organism is *Neisseria gonorrhoeae* (a Gram-negative diplococcus). Infection is by sexual contact, including oral and anal. Other means, like public lavatory seats, are little more than a theoretical possibility and usually an excuse, The incubation period is usually 2—5 days with virulent organism and low host resistance, but may be as long as 8 weeks with low virulence and high host resistance.

The sites of infection are tissues not covered with stratified squamous epithelium, i.e. commonly the urethra, including the paraurethral tubules, Bartholin's glands and the endocervix. The buccal and anal mucosa may also be involved.

CLINICAL FEATURES OF GONORRHOEA

Infected women are frequently symptomless. Otherwise the initial complaints are of dysuria, urinary frequency and vaginal discharge. The discharge causes soreness but not pruritus unless there is an associated trichomonal infection. In severe cases, the whole vulva becomes reddened and swollen; inguinal adenitis, general malaise and fever are then likely. Cystitis is a possible development. Untreated gonorrhoea persists as a chronic and contagious disease for many years. The organisms linger in the endocervix, Bartholin's glands and periurethral tubules. Remote lesions may involve joints, tendons and ligaments (probably due to associated non-gonococcal infection). Complications include endometritis, salpingitis and pelvic peritonitis. It is probably the commonest cause of tubal occlusion.

Diagnosis: This is suggested by the history of contact and the acuteness of the onset of a purulent discharge with associated urethritis and is made by demonstrating the gonococcus by Gram stain and culture. Failure to culture the organism often occurs if proper transport media and plating procedures are not used. When gonorrhoea is diagnosed or suspected it is essential to consider coexistent syphilis and to look for trichomonas which coexists in 60 per cent of cases.

TREATMENT

Penicillin   is the treatment of choice usually given as one or two large, long-acting injections to ensure that treatment is received. It is vital that contacts are followed up, and tracing contacts is a major part of any genitourinary medicine clinic.

Syphilis

Routine blood testing in antenatal clinics has led to detection of syphilis in its symptomless latent phase, which may be anything from 2 to 20 years, and a reduction in the incidence of congenital syphilis. If the disease is undetected in a pregnant woman the infant may die in utero or be born with the disease, but treatment of the infected woman in the first half of pregnancy prevents the stigmata of congenital syphilis (Hutchinson's teeth, collapsed nose, etc.). A history of fetal death should always raise the suspicion of syphilis, especially if the placenta was large.

Although much syphilis is picked up at the latent stage by antenatal screening processes, it may present in the gynaecological clinic as an ulcer on any part of the female genital tract between the vulva and cervix when the diagnosis can be made by observing the *Treponema pallidum* on dark-ground examination of exudate taken or scraped from the ulcerated lesion. The gynaecologist may also see condylomata lata, which are moist, flat warts, around the vulval area. These manifestations of secondary syphilis are usually associated with a generalized lymphadenopathy and sometimes with a non-irritative skin rash. Any such lesion should be examined with extreme care because they teem with live spirochaetes so that any examiner rash enough to approach such lesions without protective gloves may be infected through any minute abrasion in his own skin. When syphilis is diagnosed the patient should be referred to a department of genitourinary medicine, because although treatment with penicillin is usually both simple and effective, extensive investigation and prolonged follow-up is required.

Endometriosis

This is a condition in which endometrial tissue is found in ectopic sites, i.e. other than the uterine cavity.

The aetiology of endometriosis is unknown, but there are three main theories and all may be operative:

1. Implantation due to retrograde menstruation.
2. Metaplasia of coelomic derivatives.

Pelvic peritoneum and ovarian coelomic epithelium are derived embryologically from the same coelomic tissue which forms the Müllerian ducts.

3. Embolism of endometrial tissue in pelvic veins of lymphatics.

Endometriosis may affect women from their teens onwards but it is more common in the thirties and forties, in Caucasians in the so-called civilized world and is associated with sterility and low parity. It is rarer in non-Whites.

Endometriosis is oestrogen-dependent, but pregnancy leads to regression of the endometriotic tissue due to the predominance of progesterone. It does not occur before puberty and tends to regress after the menopause.

Pathology of Endometriosis

Endometrial deposits may be found in various parts of the body but are usually confined to the pelvis. The ovary is the commonest site. The pelvic peritoneum, especially in the pouch of Douglas, and the uterosacral ligaments are also frequently involved. Endometriosis may occur in the bowel, usually in the wall, resulting in stricture. If the bladder is involved cyclical haematuria may occur. Deposits of endometriosis may be found in the vagina and in scars of the abdominal wall perineum or uterus. Anterior abdominal wall scars are specially at risk if the endometrial cavity is opened, e.g. at hysterotomy or myomectomy. An endometriotic deposit at the umbilicus may cause cyclical bleeding externally. Cyclical haemoptysis as well as bleeding from the arm and leg have been reported, but these are extremely rare sites for endometriosis. The deposits of endometriosis can vary from minute pin head-sized spots coloured black by blood to large cysts filled with old altered blood which becomes thick and brown. These cysts are called 'chocolate' cysts. Since old blood in any cyst has this appearance one must see endometrial glands on microscopy to make the diagnosis of endometriosis. The ectopic endometrium bleeds when the patient menstruates since it responds to ovarian hormones as does normal endometrium. The blood can cause an intense fibrous reaction resulting in dense adhesions and cyst formation. Fibrosis is made worse if the chocolate cyst leaks or ruptures. Endometriosis is relatively commonly associated with fibroids, adenomyosis and endometrial hyperplasia.

Clinical Features of Endometriosis
The symptomatology is very variable and unrelated to the extent of the disease. The most extensive endometriosis may be asymptomatic and discovered incidentally, while small lesions may produce marked symptoms. Infertility may be the main and even only complaint. The outstanding features are deep dyspareunia and congestive dysmenorrhoea which may be caused by small deposits of endometriosis, typically in the pouch of Douglas. Menorrhagia is a frequent symptom due to vascular congestion and endometriosis of the myometrium (adenomyosis). If ovarian function is disturbed by surrounding endometriosis the cycle may also alter, usually becoming shorter.

Signs: On examination tender nodules (like lead-shot) may be felt along the uterosacral ligaments and in the pouch of Douglas due to the endometrial deposits. Tender ovarian masses may be adherent to the uterus, which may, as a result, be fixed, tender and retroverted.

Diagnosis: The differential diagnosis includes pelvic inflammatory disease, and laparoscopy should be done to confirm the diagnosis of endometriosis because clinical diagnosis is notoriously uncertain and treatment is specific and necessarily prolonged.

TREATMENT
There are two main types of treatment which may be combined: (1) hormonal and (2) surgical which may be (a) conservative or (b) radical. The choice depends on the age and parity of the patient, her desire for pregnancy and the size and extent of the lesions present.

1. *Hormonal therapy* is the treatment of choice for the younger woman with relatively small lesions and it aims at producing a 'pseudo pregnancy'. The rationale is that endometriosis improves if pregnancy occurs and goes to term. Menstruation may be suppressed for 6–9 months with (1) continuous progestogen therapy (e.g. dydrogesterone 20–30 mg daily), or (2) danazol ('danol'). This steroid suppresses gonadotrophin secretion and

thus ovarian function by negative feedback on the hypothalamus while itself having little effect on the lower genital tract. Oral treatment in a dose (200—800 mg daily) sufficient to suppress menstruation for up to 6 months is prescribed. The efficacy of any hormonal therapy may be assessed by the absence of symptomatology after therapy, by pregnancy or by repeat laparoscopy.

2a. *Conservative surgery* is indicated where fertility is desired, and discrete masses are present. Large chocolate cysts always need excision. Small endometrial deposits may be diathermized or excised. Hormonal therapy may be used in conjunction with conservative surgery.

2b. *Radical surgery* is indicated if the woman has completed her family and there are extensive masses of endometriotic tissue, cysts and adhesions present. The ovaries should be removed since any endometriotic deposits remaining will continue to bleed if ovarian function remains.

Adenomyosis (also called 'internal endometriosis')
This diagnosis is usually made histologically when endometrial tissue is found to have penetrated diffusely and deeply into the myometrium by direct extension from the lining of the endometrial cavity. The frequency with which the diagnosis is made depends on the assiduity with which the pathologist sections each uterus. Adenomyosis produces a fibrous reaction and lumps known as adenomyomas develop with many similarities to fibroids. Adenomyosis occurs most commonly in multiparous women over 30 and may be associated with fibroids, endometrial hyperplastic endometriosis and endometrial carcinoma. Endocrine imbalance (relative excess of oestrogen) is a supposed aetiological factor. The symptoms are of dysmenorrhoea, dyspareunia and menorrhagia and the signs are an enlarged and tender uterus. The differential diagnosis includes pelvic inflammatory disease, endometrial carcinoma, endometrial polyps and fibroids.

Treatment of adenomyosis is usually by hysterectomy since hormonal treatment is generally unsatisfactory.

Pelvic Pain

This is a complaint encountered with increasing frequency at the gynaecological out-patient clinic and has a variety of causes. It may be classified by the relationship to menstruation, sexual intercourse or other activity, and in other descriptive terms which help to identify the underlying cause (*see* Table 3.1).

Dysmenorrhoea
Normal menstruation in the majority of women with ovulatory cycles is associated with discomfort in the pelvis and also commonly the groins,

tops of the thighs and low back. The discomfort is of a colicky nature, most noticeable on the first day, and is aptly termed 'menstrual cramps' in North America. Most women tolerate this discomfort and only occasionally need a mild analgesic. Dysmenorrhoea is a symptom of great importance since it can cause much time off from school and work.

Primary Dysmenorrhoea

This form of dysmenorrhoea starts a year or so after the menarche when ovulatory cycles begin. It is colicky in nature, hence the term spasmodic, and is located deep in the suprapubic region, low back, groins and thighs, although not always in all sites in the same patient. Primary dysmenorrhoea

Table 3.1.   Classification of Pelvic Pain

Dysmenorrhoea   =   painful menstruation
    Primary or spasmodic
        normal cramps
        exacerbated by psychological factors
    Secondary or congestive
        Pathological
        PID
        endometriosis
        psychosexual

Dyspareunia   =   painful sexual intercourse
    Superficial
        Pathological
        infection
        post-trauma (e.g. episiotomy)
        atrophy
        Psychosexual
    Deep
        Prolapse
            ovaries in pouch of Douglas
            retroverted and retroflexed uterus in pouch of Douglas
        Pathological
        PID
        endometriosis
        cervicitis
        Psychosexual

Chronic Constant Pelvic Pain
    Pathological
        PID
    Psychosexual

Backache
    skeletal (orthopaedic) related to posture
    gynaecological related to prolapse

Iliac fossa pain
    psychosomatic
    gut, constipation, spasm

starts a few hours before or just as menstruation begins and is usually limited to the first day.

AETIOLOGY

It is essentially a severe form of 'normal' cramps and not due to any organic lesion. There is a large psychological element in many cases, and the dysmenorrhoeic mother who fails to inform her daughter about menstruation, or who hints at the 'sufferings' of women due to 'the curse' and 'being unwell' will tend to produce a dysmenorrhoeic daughter. The incidence of severe spasmodic dysmenorrhoea has decreased greatly with a more educated and sensible approach to menstruation by women. The pain is generally associated with ovulatory cycles and is produced by strong frequent uterine contractions. This hypercontractility causes painful ischaemia and may be due to an increase of prostaglandin $F_{2\alpha}$ in menstrual blood. An autonomic nervous disturbance resulting in diarrhoea is a frequent accompaniment.

TREATMENT

Treatment is most effective when ovulation is suppressed with oral contraceptive preparations. Alternatively progestogens alone may also be effective (e.g. dydrogesterone 10 mg b.d. from day 5 to day 25). In less severe cases a mild analgesic may be all that is required, but a full explanation of the condition and reassurance about normalcy should be given to all complainants. Recently success has been claimed for the use of prostaglandin synthetase inhibitors such as mefenamic acid (Ponstan; Parke-Davis) in doses of 250–500 mg thrice daily for the duration of pain.

Dilatation of the cervix carries the risk of producing cervical incompetence and its effect in pain relief is at best transient. It has no place now, nor has presacral neurectomy, which aims to denervate the uterus.

Secondary Dysmenorrhoea

This condition is so-called because it begins in adult life and is of acquired organic or psychosexual origin. It is also called 'congestive dysmenorrhoea', being thought to be associated with pelvic vascular disturbance. The pain starts many days before menstruation and gets worse as the time of menstruation approaches. It is more constant in nature and situated in the pelvis and back. It may be secondary to endometriosis or pelvic inflammatory disease and treatment is of that condition. However, laparoscopy reveals no such lesion in about half the women with congestive dysmenorrhoea and related symptoms; the condition is then called pelvic congestion syndrome (*see below*), and is often due to psychosexual problems.

Premenstrual Tension Syndrome

This is a symptom complex occurring in the week preceding menstruation, although in some patients it may occur even earlier in the cycle. It is an exaggerated form of symptoms experienced by many normal women in whom mild mood change in the 48 hours before menstruation, usually a tendency to irritability and weepiness, is common. Premenstrual tension syndrome comprises tension, irritability and depression together with a bloated feeling in the abdomen, tense, tender breasts and 'sausage' fingers. These last symptoms are due to fluid retention. The onset of the syndrome is usually in the fourth decade and is a cause of an increase in accidents, crimes and suicides at this age in the premenstrual phase.

Since it is associated with ovulatory cycles suppression of ovulation may help, or progestogens alone given in the second half of the cycle (e.g. dydrogesterone 20–40 mg daily from day 15 to day 25) may relieve the tension without suppressing ovulation. A diuretic is necessary if fluid retention is a predominant feature. Tranquillizers and antidepressants should be avoided. Psychiatric help should be sought without delay for more severe cases.

Dyspareunia

The term dyspareunia means painful intercourse. It may be due to organic or psychological causes.

Superficial Dyspareunia

This term means pain confined to the introitus. The commonest organic cause is infection, or atrophy in the older woman. An episiotomy scar may cause pain. Very rarely there is a congenital abnormality. If, on examination, patholoy is excluded, vaginismus with levator spasm and failure of the vagina to lubricate is the usual cause of such complaints as 'My vagina is too small' or 'His penis is too big'. Fear, inadequate sex education and previous painful intercourse, together with poor sexual stimulation and unskilled techniques, make for superficial dyspareunia. Education of both partners, reassurance and self-examination and a simple lubricant are all that is needed. Plastic operations and artificial dilators have no place unless an anatomical abnormality is present.

Deep Dyspareunia

The condition known as deep dyspareunia may be due to pelvic pathology, particularly endometriosis, pelvic inflammatory disease or cervicitis. In these cases the pain is felt deep in the pelvis during intercourse and usually subsides quickly after withdrawal. If the ovaries are prolapsed in the pouch of Douglas in association with a retroverted uterus, collision dyspareunia may occur due to compression of the ovaries during thrusting. The fundus of the retroverted uterus may be tender. This pain also ceases on withdrawal. Deep dyspareunia may have a psychosexual origin and in these cases often lasts 24 or 48 hours after intercourse. Nevertheless, it must not be assumed that dyspareunia lasting postcoitally is psychosexual until organic causes, especially pelvic inflammatory disease, have been excluded.

Pelvic Congestion Syndrome

The patient complains of congestive dysmenorrhoea and deep dyspareunia often together with symptoms of fluid retention similar to the premenstrual tension syndrome. There is often excessive cervical secretion leading to the complaint of vaginal discharge, lack of libido and failure to achieve orgasm. The multiplicity of complaints suggests a psychosomatic origin. Pain of psychosomatic origin rarely disturbs sleep whereas pain due to pelvic pathology may do so. Examination is often difficult, the patient refusing to relax. The uterus is usually retroverted, bulky and tender. The entire pelvis is moderately tender on examination. Having excluded endometriosis and pelvic inflammatory disease by laparoscopy, psychosexual counselling with attention to contraception is needed. Hysterectomy may be required in the last resort, when congested pelvic veins and thickened fibrosed uterosacral ligaments may be found. The bulky uterus will look mottled but histologically reveal no abnormality. Pelvic pain may continue even after total hysterectomy and bilateral salpingo-oophorectomy, and the psychologically pain-dependent patient must be recognized before being subjected to unnecessary gynaecological procedures. Laparoscopic exclusion of serious organic disease may be sufficient to relieve symptoms in some anxious patients.

Backache

Low backache may be of gynaecological origin related to menstruation, pelvic pathology and psychosexual problems, but the majority of back pains are due to disorders of the back and the help of an orthopaedic surgeon should be sought. Backache due to musculoskeletal disorders is commonly related to bending and lifting and is often worse at night due to poor bed-support. It is not related to menstruation but can seem worse before periods due to subjective changes associated with the premenstrual part of the cycle. A mobile retroversion of the uterus is a normal asymptomatic finding in 25 per cent of women and does not cause backache. The early but not the late stages of prolapse may be associated with low backache, worse on standing and relieved by recumbancy.

Iliac Fossa Pain

Chronic constipation, spasm of the descending colon and back pressure on the caecum causing gaseous distension are common causes. Constipation is common in females and should not be discounted even if the patient has regular bowel actions. A tender loaded colon is palpable in the left iliac fossa, a gurgling distended caecum in the right. The patient should eat a high fibre diet including fresh vegetables, fruit and bran, and take plenty of fluids. Occasionally iliac fossa pain can be associated with ovarian or tubal pathology.

Chapter four

Retroversion, Prolapse and Urinary Problems

RETROVERSION

In childhood the uterus is a straight upright organ, its body being small in relation to the cervix. As the uterus grows at puberty the body enlarges to a greater extent than the cervix and usually leans forward upon it causing both angulation of the body on the cervix (anteflexion) and rotation of the whole uterus forward on its supporting ligaments (anteversion). However, the uterus is a mobile active organ contracting throughout reproductive life and can take up many positions. The position of the uterus is altered by changes in adjacent organs particularly the bladder as it fills and empties. During intercourse in the late excitement phase the uterus is elevated, thus effectively lengthening the vagina. The uterus may be pushed backwards by a mass of fibroids growing from its anterior wall, or forwards by a tumour, usually an ovarian cyst, occupying the pouch of Douglas. A cyst growing from the left ovary may displace the uterus to the right, whereas left adnexal inflammatory disease may draw the uterus across to the left. Although the uterus usually lies in an anteverted, ante-flexed position when the bladder is empty, in 25 per cent of women it will be retroverted (but not usually retroflexed). This retroverted position may be quite normal provided the uterus is mobile and it usually presents no problems. Retroversion may be acquired due to pelvic inflammatory disease or endometriosis in which case it is fixed and cannot be corrected.

Mobile ('Congenital') Retroversion

This is usually asymptomatic, and it is necessary to assess any symptomatology very carefully before attributing it to a mobile retroverted uterus. Backache due to congestion of the uterus as a result of impaired venous drainage may sometimes occur, but backache is much more commonly due to other conditions. Dyspareunia means painful intercourse. Deep dyspareunia, that is pain felt deep in the pelvis at the top of the vagina during intercourse, may occur if the ovaries are prolapsed in the pouch of Douglas. Dysmenorrhoea, that is pain due to menstruation, is not related to mobile retroversion, and mobile retroversion is not a cause of infertility.

Fixed acquired retroversion is due to pathology, usually pelvic inflammatory disease or endometriosis, which are discussed in Chapter 3. The symptoms, signs and management depend on the underlying disease but backache, deep dyspareunia, dysmenorrhoea and infertility may all be present with fixed retroversion, being caused by the basic pathology causing the retroversion to be fixed.

Retroversion in Pregnancy

When a patient with a mobile retroverted uterus becomes pregnant the uterus fills the pelvis by 12 weeks, becoming anteverted and easily palpable abdominally by 14 weeks. If the uterus is prevented from rising out of the pelvis by adhesions, impaction and incarceration may occur, leading to abortion. This set of events is heralded by urinary disturbance, first frequency, then strangury and finally retention. Acute retention in the female is a rare event and is due to a retroverted uterus enlarged by pregnancy and/or tumour (usually ovarian or fibromyomatous) to the size of a 14-week pregnancy being impacted in the pelvis, distorting and compressing the bladder neck. Before the menarche a haematocolpos (a uterus filled with blood) can cause acute retention. Other rare causes are urethral trauma and neurological damage.

The diagnosis of retroversion is made on bimanual examination. The differential diagnosis is from other masses in the pouch of Douglas; the passage of a sound will define the position of the uterus if confusion persists. To determine whether symptoms are directly referable to the retroversion a Hodge pessary test is done. This involves placing a Hodge pessary after correction of the retroversion in the vagina to hold the uterus in anteversion for a few weeks. If the symptoms are relieved, surgical correction of the retroversion (ventrosuspension) is likely to be successful. If the retroversion is mobile, manipulation to an anteverted position alone is pointless since the mobile retroverted uterus will return to its usual position. Ventrosuspension involves shortening the round ligaments and suturing them to the rectus sheath, and may be done at laparotomy or laparoscopy. Plication of the round ligaments alone holds the uterus forward temporarily and is often done as an adjunct to surgery for some other condition to avoid postoperative adhesions binding the uterus down in the pouch of Douglas.

PROLAPSE

The remarkable thing about uterine prolapse in the human is not that it occurs commonly but that it is not universal. Since woman (or her ancestors) assumed the erect posture the weight of pelvic and abdominal contents has to be supported across an aperture which is large enough to allow the passage of a baby. Obviously the supporting mechanism must be sufficiently elastic to allow this passage to occur. Phylogenetically woman has achieved this by converting the muscles used by her predecessors to wag their tails into a muscular hammock across the pelvis. This hammock is formed of the levator ani muscles, which are the main support of the vagina acting through their insertion into the perineal body. The main supports of the uterus and vaginal vault are the various condensations of the pelvic fascia especially the transverse cervical ligaments (*see* Chapter 2.)

Definition: Prolapse is the downward eversion of a hollow organ towards or out of its introitus (or extroitus) and may involve the rectum, vagina or urethra. (For information regarding rectal prolapse the student is referred to a textbook of surgery.)

Vaginal Wall Prolapse

A prolapse of the lowest third of the anterior vaginal wall involves the urethra and is called a urethrocoele. A prolapse of the upper two-thirds of the anterior vaginal wall is a cystocoele, since bladder is involved. A prolapse of the pouch of Douglas is an enterocoele, and the peritoneal sac of the enterocoele may contain gut, omentum, appendix and virtually any other lower abdominal organ. Prolapse of the posterior wall of the vagina is termed a rectocoele and is distinct from rectal prolapse where the rectal mucosa extrudes through the anus turning the rectum inside out. A rectocoele is a slipping forwards of the rectum into the vagina and through the introitus pushing the posterior vaginal wall in front of it.

Uterine Prolapse (Vault Prolapse)

The uterus may prolapse on its own, but usually there is concomitant vaginal wall prolapse. Conversely the vaginal wall may prolapse without uterine or vault descent. Uterine prolapse is divided into three degrees:

First degree descent occurs when the cervix and uterus move down the vagina below the ischial spines.

Second degree descent occurs when the cervix protrudes through the introitus.

Third degree descent, or procidentia, has occurred when the uterus lies entirely outside the introitus.

Aetiology

Disturbance of the support mechanisms leading to prolapse may occur due to: (1) childbirth, (2) oestrogen deficiency (postmenopausal atrophy) or (3) chronically raised intra-abdominal pressure.

Prolapse is more common in parous women, particularly those who have had difficult deliveries. Destruction of the perineum and pelvic floor mechanism following difficult or repeated childbirth, or inadequate repair of episiotomy or tear, leave a gaping introitus with the anterior vaginal wall unsupported. This slips down and the uterus, whose ligaments may have been excessively stretched during delivery, descends too. While it is common to see some element of prolapse in many patients early in the puerperium after normal confinement due to stretching of the perineum and laxity of the pelvic floor, most patients have recovered their pelvic floor tone by 3 months. However, most parous women have some laxity of the anterior vaginal wall in particular and some degree of perineal deficiency.

Prolapse usually presents in the peri- and postmenopausal years, the delay being due to the additional factor of oestrogen deficiency. This affects the strength of the cardinal and uterosacral ligaments, as well as the uterus, vaginal skin and subcutaneous tissue of the external genitalia, and loss of muscle tone in the pelvis and elsewhere.

Raised intra-abdominal pressure stresses the supports of the uterus and vagina, and the mechanism of urinary continence (*see below*), in the acute situation (e.g. coughing, laughing, sneezing, etc.) and in the chronic situation. It is the latter which helps to produce prolapse. The obese patient, with a chronic cough from smoking or bronchitis, who strains at stool and has done so for years because of constipation has a chronically stressed pelvic floor. Large pelvic tumours may also be a contributing factor. Many patients with prolapse exhibit one or more of these features which are best corrected before surgical repair is undertaken.

Clinical Features

The typical patient is a parous postmenopausal woman who complains of 'something coming down', or of stress incontinence. The patient may be aware of a lump protruding from the vulva or simply of a feeling of insecurity and downward pressure. Occasionally prolapse is seen in younger women immediately following delivery or, very rarely, during pregnancy. It is also less common in Negresses and Asians, possibly because of their customary training as girls to develop their pelvic floor muscles (probably mainly for sexual performance).

Pain is not a feature, but backache sometimes occurs and is characteristically worse at the end of the day and relieved by rest. Bleeding due to prolapse is rare and should only be attributed to the prolapse after thorough investigation including curettage.

In cases of chronic procidentia there is vascular stasis. The vaginal skin is atrophic, poor perfusion of the tissues increases the vulnerability of the tissues and ulceration due to friction of underclothing is not uncommon.

Stress incontinence, that is leakage of urine when intra-abdominal pressure is raised with coughing, sneezing or movement, may occur in the absence of anterior vaginal wall prolapse but is a complaint frequently found in association with a cystourethrocoele (*see* section on urinary problems).

Urinary retention and sometimes difficulty with defaecation occasionally occur and may be relieved by the patient pushing the prolapse back into the vagina herself. Many patients with prolapse, some with procidentia, have no complaints, the prolapse being an incidental finding.

With virginal (nulliparous or telescopic) prolapse the primary defect is a weakness of the ligamentous supports of the uterus due to oestrogen deficiency. Because of their weakness the uterus becomes axial to the vagina and the cervix descends to a lower level in the vagina. As the descent of uterus and cervix continues the vaginal walls are peeled off the subjacent structures and eventually the vagina may be completely everted but the perineum is intact. Once the uterus and cervix are restored to their normal position, however, there is no cystocoele or rectocoele to be found.

Examination and demonstration of prolapse is best carried out with the patient in the left lateral position using a Sims speculum to hold back the posterior vaginal wall and a sponge forceps to hold back the anterior vaginal wall, although a procidentia will be apparent in whatever position the patient lies. Inspection of the introitus while the patient coughs may reveal stress incontinence, a urethrocoele, cystocoele and rectocoele. The cervix may become visible too. Examination should be carried out in a systematic manner to observe the various parts that may contribute to prolapse. As all parts of the vaginal skin are seen, an assessment of its oestrogenization is made. First the lower third of the anterior wall is viewed for a urethrocoele, then the upper two-thirds. The patient may be asked to cough or bear down. The degree of mobility and descent of the uterus and cervix can very well be assessed bimanually, but a single-toothed Volsellum may be applied to the cervix which can then be drawn down to demonstrate the degree of uterine prolapse. As this often causes the patient discomfort, which is marked in some cases, and may yield little helpful information regarding management, we have almost abandoned it and rely on careful bimanual assessment of uterine mobility and descent.

It is important to view the posterior fornix, particularly as the patient coughs, but it can often be very difficult to demonstrate an enterocoele. As the speculum is withdrawn it is possible to see the posterior vaginal wall bulge forwards, and the rectocoele and perineal integrity may be demonstrated by placing a finger in the rectum and gently pushing the anterior rectal wall against the posterior vaginal wall. The bulge of the rectocoele will be seen at the introitus. Combined rectovaginal examination after removal of the speculum may help, particularly when trying to detect an enterocoele.

Treatment

Although prolapse is not life threatening and may be asymptomatic, in the majority of cases it causes misery, alters the patient's life style, restricts her activity and requires treatment. Before deciding which form of treatment is appropriate a careful assessment should be made paying particular attention to the following features:

1. The patient's age and parity, especially the wish for more children.
2. Sexual activity and the need for a functional vagina.
3. The presence of aggravating factors such as obesity and smoking,

which should be eliminated before surgery. Their elimination improves the efficacy of conservative treatment too.

4. Menstrual problems.
5. Urinary symptoms, which must be carefully analysed.

Prophylactic

Proper attention to the repair of the perineum and avoiding overstretching of perineum during delivery, together with regular postnatal pelvic floor exercises will help prevent prolapse. Avoidance of those factors chronically raising intra-abdominal pressure and the judicious use of oestrogen therapy at the menopause may also prevent prolapse.

Conservative

If a patient wants more children, or is unfit for surgery; if there is a long waiting-list or she is attending the dietician, it is often possible to control the prolapse and alleviate the symptoms using a pessary. The common type is a ring pessary. These come in different sizes and are made of plastic. Rings should be changed at regular 3—4 monthly intervals. They should be washed before replacement and the vagina inspected to exclude any trauma. Rings are only satisfactory for lesser degrees of prolapse. In the postmenopausal woman an oestrogen cream should be used once or twice a week to prevent atrophy. There are other sorts of pessary, the shelf and stem and the cup and stem, but these are rarely used. They are used when a ring fails to control the prolapse. Shelf pessaries give satisfactory control of major prolapse but make coitus impossible and are difficult to fit. Physiotherapy to the pelvic floor muscles, including faradism, and to the chest for patients with chronic bronchitis, together with weight loss, may cure stress incontinence, or be useful adjuncts to a pessary or preparation for surgery.

Surgery

PREOPERATIVE PREPARATION

It is important to define and eradicate, where possible, contributory factors. For instance the obese patient should be encouraged to lose weight. Overweight patients are an operative hazard in any field of surgery. She should stop smoking for at least 3 months before surgery, and chest physiotherapy may be helpful. Constipation should be eradicated. Local oestrogen creams improve the quality of vaginal skin, and ulcers should be healed before surgery. Prolapse has never killed a patient but surgical repair of prolapse has, so for this elective procedure, which is carried out for the patient's comfort rather than immediate health, she should be as fit as possible. The chance of recurrence of the prolapse postoperatively is also reduced.

CHOICE OF OPERATION

The type of operation carried out depends on what is involved in the prolapse. For instance anterior vaginal wall repair is appropriate for a cystocoele; posterior colpoperineorrhaphy (repair) for a rectocoele. If there is uterine (i.e. vaginal vault) prolapse the vault may be best repaired if the uterus is coincidentally removed (vaginal hysterectomy and repair).

Alternatively the uterus and vault may be supported by shortening the transverse cervical ligaments, which necessitates partial cervical amputation; when combined with anterior and posterior colpoperineorrhaphy as is often necessary, the whole procedure is called the Manchester (or Fothergill) Repair Operation. Many gynaecologists now favour vaginal hysterectomy and repair because the long-term results in terms of recurrent prolapse are better, the patients are rarely young – and even the younger patients usually desire foolproof contraception, and in any case child-bearing after cervical amputation can be hazardous.

URINARY PROBLEMS

The Mechanisms of Continence and Micturition

Urinary problems present commonly to the gynaecologist. They may be associated with prolapse or other gynaecological disorders and since they date from childbearing the patient seeks gynaecological rather than urological advice. An understanding of the mechanisms of continence and micturition aids successful treatment, but they have long been an enigma and the subject is still surrounded by controversy. Recently the use of urodynamic studies, namely of urethral and vesical pressure, urine flow, and cineradiographic visualization of the changes taking place during micturition, have led to the mechanisms being defined more accurately.

Continence

There are three muscular components (or 'sphincters') which help keep the urethra closed and empty except during voiding. These three components certainly function as sphincters but there is no accumulation of circular muscle as, for instance, at the pylorus.

1. The innermost component is situated at the bladder neck and is of fundamental importance. It is composed of parts of the detrusor muscle, the main part of which actually opens the bladder neck to initiate micturition. Some smooth muscle bundles are inserted into the trigone and pull the apex of the trigone forward. The net effect of these two sets of fibres is to keep the bladder neck and proximal urethra closed and the bladder base flat. The proximal urethra is intra-abdominal. The bladder neck only functions as a sphincter as long as the bladder base remains flat and the proximal urethra closed and subject to intra-abdominal pressure, so that a distinct angle is made at the urethrovesical junction. When normal voiding takes place the bladder base descends and the proximal urethra opens, the

bladder neck thus becoming cone- or funnel-shaped and the urethrovesical angle flattening out.

2. The urethral wall contains circularly looping smooth muscle fibres within connective tissue, which also includes much elastic tissue.

3. The external sphincter is formed by the voluntary striated muscles at the level of the urogenital diaphragm and the innermost fibres of the levator ani.

In the resting state these three muscular components exert pressure. The intraurethral pressure always exceeds the intravesical pressure, which is low, and the urethra is kept closed. The urethral closing pressure is distributed along its entire length but maximally at its mid-position. A cough or strain which increases intra-abdominal pressure, raises both intravesical and intraurethral pressure equally in a normal person, thus maintaining adequate closing pressure.

Micturition

Just before micturition begins, the intraurethral pressure falls. As micturition starts the detrusor contracts, the electrical activity passing from the dome of the bladder to the bladder neck pulling open the bladder neck; the bladder base becomes funnel-shaped, and when intravesical pressure exceeds intraurethral pressure the closing pressure becomes inadequate and urine enters the urethra.

During voiding, the detrusor continues to contract, but both smooth and striated muscles of the urethra are inactive. At the end of micturition, or if voiding is interrupted voluntarily, the flow is cut off first at the level of the external sphincter, and the urine remaining in the posterior urethra is 'milked-back' into the bladder.

The innervation of the bladder and the smooth muscle of the urethra is autonomic. Preganglionic parasympathetic fibres from S2, 3 and 4 provide the main motor supply to the detrusor. The function of the sympathetic fibres from T11 to L2 coming via the hypogastric nerves and pelvic plexus is controversial. They carry afferent impulses (especially pain), and it is suggested that they produce relaxation of the proximal urethra at the start of micturition. The striated muscle of the 'external sphincter', that is the muscles at the level of the urogenital diaphragm including the innermost fibres of the levator ani, are supplied by the pudendal nerve.

Micturition is controlled by a spinal reflex which can be inhibited or facilitated by impulses from the cortex and other higher centres or facilitated by perineal stimulation.

Urinary Incontinence

Urinary incontinence is a common symptom presented to the gynaecologist and has a number of very different causes which can be distinguished to a large extent by the exact mode of presentation.

Type	Causes
Stress	Bladder neck incompetence
Urge	Infection
	Unstable bladder
Continuous	Retention with overflow
	Fistula

Stress Incontinence

This is defined as involuntary loss of urine when the intra-abdominal pressure is raised, as by coughing, laughing, sneezing, etc., in the absence of any desire to void. True stress incontinence is caused by incompetence of the sphincteric mechanism at the bladder neck (component 1) which allows the bladder base to funnel and allows the proximal part of the urethra to descend outside the abdominal cavity. The patient thus depends on the other two muscular components to maintain continence, that is the urethral wall and the (voluntary) external sphincter; whilst they maintain continence at rest they cannot withstand a 'stress' of raised intra-abdominal pressure, so urine leaks. Typical urodynamic findings in a patient with defective bladder neck sphincter are that the bladder is of normal capacity and that the pressure remains low during filling. The urethral closing pressure is low and cannot be greatly increased when the patient tries to 'squeeze' the measuring device. When the patient coughs, urine leaks in the absence of a detrusor contraction. Urine is voided at a normal rate but the stream cannot be interrupted.

Urgency and Urge Incontinence

Urinary urgency is the intense desire to void, which, if overwhelming, leads to incontinence, hence called urge incontinence. There are two distinct types. *Sensory urgency* occurs commonly in inflammatory bladder diseases and is rarely associated with incontinence. *Motor urgency* is followed by incontinence as it is caused by detrusor contraction.

The Unstable Bladder

It has been observed that detrusor contractions can occur involuntarily and cause incontinence. The condition has various names: unstable bladder, uninhibited bladder and detrusor dyssynergia. The patient complains of frequency but may also complain of urgency and urge and stress incontinence.

It is detected on urodynamic examination by spikes of increased intravesical pressure causing leakage which may occur spontaneously during bladder filling (or when the patient coughs), and the bladder capacity is functionally reduced. The sphincters of such a patient will be normal and thus the urethral closing pressure will be normal.

If the patient is leaking urine continuously the following causes must be investigated.

Chronic Retention with Overflow
A small percentage of incontinent women, particularly those who have
previously undergone a repair operation, will be found to have outflow
obstruction, situated commonly in the distal urethra and rarely at the
bladder neck. They will have a large capacity bladder, high urethral
resistance and a low flow rate, and are usually asymptomatic. A further
small group with neuropathy (mainly diabetics) have deficient detrusor
function and therefore are functionally obstructed as they have a very low
flow rate in the presence of normal urethral resistance.

Fistulae
The ureter or bladder may communicate with the uterus or vagina and the
patient will have no control over the urinary flow. Fistulae follow radiotherapy, advanced malignant disease and surgery or primitive obstetrics.
Rarely an ectopic ureter may open in to the vagina.

Clinical Presentation
Stress and urge incontinence are the commonest types of incontinence and
often occur together and in varying degree. It is important to appreciate
that stress incontinence occurs to a slight degree in 10—15 per cent of all
normal women, especially after the menopause, and surgery is an excessive
measure to take in such cases.

On the other hand the incontinence may be so severe that urine soaks
through outer layers of clothes causing such embarrassment and misery as
to imprison the patient in her home. Typically the patient is postmenopausal and parous. A detailed enquiry must always be made about
the exact circumstances under which leakage occurs and to elicit any other
urinary symptoms such as dysuria, frequency (diurnal passage of urine at
less than 2-hourly intervals) and nocturia (waking from sleep to void).
Other important points are, of course, a full obstetric and gynaecological
history and a story of any previous operation or irradiation, neurological
lesion, diabetes, urinary infection or childhood eneuresis.

Clinical examination is relatively unrewarding, as although virtually all
parous women have some degree of vaginal wall laxity, stress incontinence
can occur without any prolapse. If a cystourethrocoele is present then the
bladder and urethra have distended and the base-plate will be distorted
from its normal flat shape and will adopt the funnel shape seen in patients
at the onset of voiding. When a very large cystocoele is present the bladder
base can again become flat and this correlates with the clinical observation
that an enormous cystocoele often does not cause incontinence.

Treatment
Surgical repair in instances where the patient has leakage only on stress
(coughing, laughing, sneezing, walking, running, etc.) is indicated and
produces satisfactory results. However, if the patient complains of fre-

quency or nocturia, or urgency and urge incontinence, it is very likely that the bladder is unstable, and whether or not a prolapse is present, patients with an unstable bladder will not benefit from repair operation. Their incontinence is not improved after operation, but treatment with emepronium bromide 200 mg (Cetiprin; KabiVitrum) may help by blocking peripheral cholinergic nerves and ganglionic transmission to increase bladder capacity. The distinction between stress incontinence and unstable bladder can often only be made satisfactorily by urodynamic investigation, and infection should be excluded in every patient with urinary symptoms.

Further Reading

Stanton S. L. (ed.) (1978) *Gynaecological Urology. Clinics in Obstetrics and Gynaecology*, 5(1). Eastbourne, Saunders.

Chapter five

Abnormal Vaginal Bleeding

This chapter is orientated to the clinical problems of abnormal vaginal bleeding because it is a very common symptom with a wide variety of causes, including carcinoma, and the differential diagnosis is of great practical importance. The individual causes are described in other chapters. Abnormal vaginal bleeding may be classified into:

1. Abnormal menstrual bleeding
   a. Excessive
   b. Reduced
   c. Inappropriate (by age)
2. Non-menstrual bleeding.

A careful history can usually distinguish between menstrual and non-menstrual bleeding. The distinction is of great importance because, while menstrual disorders invariably have benign causes that originate beyond the endometrium, non-menstrual bleeding is often from a local lesion, commonly a carcinoma of endometrium or cervix which must therefore be urgently sought. Menstrual bleeding is recognized by the typical loss (even when excessive it occurs in a typical pattern, uninterrupted for a few days with an early peak) and by its cyclicity (even when the cycle is irregular), whereas non-menstrual bleeding is non-cyclical and patternless. When in doubt one should assume the worse, i.e. non-menstrual bleeding.

Abnormal Menstrual Bleeding
Abnormal menstrual bleeding can easily be classified and defined in its various forms given the definition of normal menstruation (*see* Chapter 1).

Excessive Menstrual Bleeding
Excessive Menses but Normal Cycle ('Menorrhagia')
The blood lost in the menses is excessive enough to clot, and necessitates the use of towels rather than tampons and in excessive number. The duration of loss may or may not be prolonged. The actual blood lost at each menstruation, although of course not measured in practice, is regularly more than 80 ml. The causes to consider are:

Fibroids
  (Chapter 6)
Ovarian endocrine disorder
  ('dysfunctional bleeding')   } Painless
Coagulation defects
  (rare)
Pelvic inflammation or adhesions
  (Chapter 3)
Endometriosis   } Painful (i.e. congestive
  (Chapter 3)   dysmenorrhoea and deep
Sexual dysfunction   dyspareunia: *see* Chapter 3)
  (Chapter 7)

Short Cycle (<21 Days) but Normal Menses ('Epimenorrhoea' or 'Poly-menorrhoea')
These cycles are always anovular and due to disorder of the ovarian endocrine axis.

Short Cycle and Excessive Menses ('Epimenorrhagia')
The causes are those responsible for menorrhagia or epimenorrhoea. Ovarian dysfunction is implied in all cases but is commonly secondary to vascular congestion due to extraovarian lesions.

Excessive Menses at Long Intervals
The typical cause is anovular ovarian disorder in which there is prolonged oestrogen porduction. The effect on the endometrium, unopposed by progesterone, results in cystic hyperplasia of the endometrium. This syndrome is called 'metropathia haemorrhagica'. However, in many cases the typical endometrial hyperplasia is absent; indeed secretory changes due to progesterone may be present. Thus the all-embracing term of 'ovarian endocrine dysfunction' (or 'dysfunctional bleeding') is generally used.

'Dysfunctional Bleeding' (Due to Ovarian Endocrine Disorder)
Ovarian disorder (strictly disorder of the hypothalamic-pituitary-ovarian axis) results in menstrual abnormality, because the endometrium is generally merely a slave to the endocrine signals it receives. The disorder particularly affects the length of the menstrual cycle. The bleeding may, however, be totally disordered and patternless, but in those cases a local lesion must be carefully excluded first. The endocrine disorder can be proven by the absence or deficiency of progesterone. However, these conditions have been imperfectly studied, and in clinical practice there is no use in endocrine determinations unless infertility is an associated problem. Indeed, because these disorders commonly occur in the early and late menstrual years, contraception is the more frequent associated need.

Diagnosis and Treatment of Excessive Menstrual Bleeding

An accurate history is essential (see above). Pelvic tumours and tenderness must be sought and treated appropriately (see Chapters 3 and 6). If the pelvic organs feel normal the diagnosis is dysfunctional bleeding and is confirmed if there is a normal menstrual response to hormone therapy (see below). Diagnostic curettage is unnecessary and unhelpful in most cases. It usually only needs to be done if hormone treatment is unsuccessful or contraindicated to search for an endometrial lesion. Coagulation disorders are rare causes of menorrhagia and need only be investigated if there is a specific lead given in the history, such as easy bruising or a familial association.

Treatment depends on the nature of any causative lesion and on the wishes of the patient, including her associated desire for contraception or pregnancy. She may be satisfied merely to know that the condition is harmless. Menstrual disorders resulting in anaemia always need treatment.

Dysfunctional bleeding is most reliably controlled with combined oestrogen and progestogen oral contraception preparations (see Chapter 8). When bleeding is heavy a preparation containing a relatively large progestogen dose is sometimes necessary (e.g. as in Gynovlar or Anovlar). Many patients resume normal menstruation after the treatment is stopped, and treatment should, therefore, be limited initially to only 2–3 cycles – unless, of course, it is also to be used to provide for contraception.

If oestrogen therapy is contraindicated (see Chapter 8), then progestogen given alone in the second half of the cycle, days 15–25, is effective in about half the cases (e.g. norethisterone acetate 5–10 mg daily). Alternatively drugs that modify capillary integrity (e.g. ethamsylate) or fibrinolysis (e.g. epsilon-aminocaproic acid) will be partially helpful in half the cases. Hysterectomy is always available as a last resort, but the patient's sometimes fervent desire for the operation may hide psychological or sexual problems that need to be properly explored.

Reduced Menstrual Bleeding

Unlike excessive menstrual bleeding, reduced bleeding is often due to endocrine disorder of serious origin, and frequently occurs in the middle reproductive years when pregnancy is desired, so that proper endocrinological investigations are needed. Thus they are mainly dealt with in Chapter 10. However, they are classified as follows:

Scanty Menstrual Bleeding ('Hypomenorrhoea')

The loss usually amounts to no more than a smear lasting not more than 2 days. It is occasionally a normal variant but most commonly occurs in association with infrequent menstrual periods (oligomenorrhoea) as a result of infrequent and impaired ovarian follicular maturation and oestrogen production. Rarely it is due to endometrial scarring and partial obliteration of the endometrial cavity (Asherman's syndrome) following traumatic curettage after abortion or childbirth.

Infrequent Menstrual Periods ('Oligomenorrhoea'): see Chapter 10.
Absent Menstrual Periods ('Amenorrhoea'): see Chapter 10.

Inappropriate Menstrual Bleeding
Menstrual bleeding is abnormal before the age of 10 years ('precocious puberty': *see* Chapter 9), after 60 years ('delayed menopause') or more than 6 months after a normal menopause. In the last case the isolated resurgence of ovarian activity may be normal, but it is usually impossible to distinguish with certainty from bleeding due to endometrial carcinoma, so that diagnostic curettage is necessary. With delayed menopause there is some concern about possible endometrial carcinoma due to prolonged (albeit cyclical) oestrogen stimulation unopposed by progesterone, anovulation being presumed. Although the risk is doubtful, curettage is a wise precaution.

Non-Menstrual Bleeding
This is non-cyclical, patternless vaginal bleeding which is usually referred to, purely descriptively, as 'postcoital' (PCB), 'intermenstrual' (IMB) or 'postmenopausal' (PMB). IMB and PMB are mutually exclusive, obviously, but either may occur in addition to PCB. (The term 'metrorrhagia' is often used for non-menstrual bleeding but is an inappropriate choice because its meaning — uterine bleeding — is too general.) The implication of non-menstrual bleeding is an anatomical lesion, which must be assumed to be a carcinoma until proved otherwise. Bleeding after coital contact suggests a cervical rather than endometrial lesion whereas IMB or PMB suggests the reverse, but this is not an infallible guide. The causes to consider are shown in Table 5.1.

Non-menstrual bleeding is not always due to a lesion. Indeed the commonest cause in young women is abortion (Chapter 11), which will be suggested by preceding amenorrhoea and perhaps pain. Ovarian endocrine disorder sometimes causes totally irregular or prolonged 'dysfunctional' bleeding. Oral contraceptives, particularly the progestogen-only pill, sometimes fail to inhibit properly endometrial bleeding, which is then called 'break-through bleeding' Chapter 8).

Investigation
Non-menstrual bleeding always requires investigation. This involves inspection, diagnostic curettage and, if there is a visible lesion, biopsy. Remember that cytology is no substitute for careful visualization of the cervix, because false negative cytology is commoner with invasive carcinoma than intraepithelial carcinoma, which is symptomless in any case. Diagnostic curettage (but not inspection) can reasonably be postponed in young

Table 5.1.   Causes of non-menstrual bleeding

Site	Cause	Comments	Chapter Reference
Vulva	Carcinoma	usually postmenopausal	6
Vagina	Vaginitis		
	infective		3
	atrophic		9
	Carcinoma		6
	squamous		
	adeno-	rare but often adolescent	
Cervix	Mucosal ectopy ('erosion')		
	Ectropion		} 6
	Cervicitis		3
	Polyps	common at all ages	
	Carcinoma		
	squamous	top priority at all ages	} 6
	adeno-		
Uterine body	Abortion	common	
	IUCD	common	} 8
	Endometrial polyps		
	Endometrial hyperplasia		
	Endometrial carcinoma	top priority after menopause	} 6
	Choriocarcinoma		
Fallopian tubes	Carcinoma		6
Ovaries	Oestrogenic tumours		6
	Dysfunction		
	('dysfunctional bleeding')	common	5
Exogenous hormones	Oral contraceptives		
	('break-through bleeding')	common	8
	Oestrogen replacement		9

women when the bleeding has lasted less than a month. Dysfunctional or break-through bleeding may persist throughout a disordered cycle and need only be considered if it occurs in more than one cycle.

The finding on diagnostic curettage of proliferative endometrium after the menopause necessitates looking at the ovaries for an oestrogen-secreting tumour if there has not been exogenous oestrogen administration to account for it.

When bleeding persists after an abortion or childbirth for more than 6 weeks the possibility of a choriocarcinoma should never be overlooked. Although rare it is truly curable.

Treatment

The treatment is of the cause — *see* the appropriate chapter reference in Table 5.1

Chapter six

Genital Neoplasia and Tumours

General

Prevalence and Incidence

Cancer, i.e. any invasive malignant tumour, occurs nearly as often in women (48·5 per cent) as in men (51·5 per cent). Table 6.1 shows that while cancer of the alimentary tract occurs equally in men and women, men are much more likely to have lung cancer, and women to have cancer of the breast or genital tract. The likelihood of cancer occurring in a

Table 6.1. Proportionate incidence (percentage) of the main sites of origin of cancer in women compared with men

Site	Women	Men
Alimentary	27	29
Lungs	5	31
Breast	25	0·2
Genital	18	9
Others	–	–
Totals	100	100

woman during her life-time is about 21 per cent, and in a man 23 per cent. Cancer of the breast alone will occur in about 5 per cent of women, and of the genital tract in 4 per cent.

In general, the risk of cancer increases with age. It is rare before 30 years, but thereafter in women the age-specific incidence increases linearly; it accelerates later in men and at about 55 years overtakes the rate in women. The general, i.e. linear, pattern in women applies to cancer of the breast, but not the genital tract. *Fig.* 6.1 shows that the greatest risk of endometrial or ovarian cancer is in the first two decades after the menopause and then falls, whereas the risk of cervical cancer is at a constant high level from about 10 years before the menopause. At the age of 40 years a woman is about four times more likely to have cervical than endometrial or ovarian cancer. From 55 years the risk is about the same

71

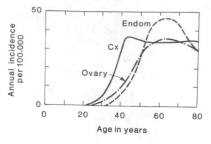

Fig. 6.1. The age-specific incidence of cancer (invasive malignant tumours) in the common sites in the genital tract: cervix (Cx), endometrium (Endom) and ovary.

Table 6.2.   Incidence, prevalent age, survival and proportion of deaths in women due to breast and genital cancer, and preinvasive cervical carcinoma

Site	Life-time incidence* (% of women)	Cause as % of all deaths	Mean age (yr)	Age range (95% limits) (yr)	5-year survival rate† (%)
Breast	5·11	3·94	60	35–86	49
Genital (total)	3·72	2·68	59	34–84	44
Cervix	1·29	0·74	55	33–84	44
Endometrium	1·02	0·37	61	41–83	70
Ovary	0·97	1·24	58	31–82	26
Vulva	0·21	0·15	67	36–89	52
Cervix preinvasive	?	–	42	25–66	~100

*Calculated from average observed annual age-specific incidence rates and 74-yr life expectancy.
†Survival rate corrected to allow for deaths not due to cancer.

for all three sites. *Fig.* 6.1 and Table 6.2 show that although endometrial cancer is rare before about the age of 40 years, ovarian cancer is not uncommon between 30 and 40 years.

Table 6.2 also shows that preinvasive (squamous) carcinoma of the cervix occurs at a mean age (which is also the peak age of incidence) about 13 years earlier than invasive cancer. This suggests that the natural progression from preinvasive to invasive carcinoma of the cervix takes about this length of time.

Cancer in other parts of the genital tract is much less common than in the cervix, endometrium or ovary (Table 6.2). Cancer of the vulva is next in frequency and occurs in the UK about 10 years later. Cancer of the vagina, Fallopian tube or myometrium, or choriocarcinoma, is extremely rare.

These data are mainly derived from an English midland population of about 5 million in the 1960s (*see* Waterhouse, 1974).

Death and Survival Rates

About 20 per cent of women die from cancer, and about 23 per cent of men. Amongst women who die from cancer, the tumour originates in the breast in 20 per cent and the genital tract in 14 per cent. These figures for breast and genital tract are lower than their relative incidence (Table 6.1) because survival is generally better than, for instance, alimentary cancer. Table 6.2 shows, however, that while survival from endometrial cancer is particularly good, that from ovarian cancer is particularly bad. The difference is at least partly due to the relatively early occurrence of symptoms with endometrial cancer (vaginal bleeding).

Towards Earlier Diagnosis

The chance of survival is greatly improved by treatment at an early stage. Early diagnosis will be the main concern of the non-specialist. The opportunity is unfortunately often missed, for various reasons:

1. Ovarian tumours are commonly asymptomatic. They should always be sought by bimanual pelvic examination whenever vaginal examination is done for other reasons, such as to take a cervical smear, to fit a contraceptive device or at the first antenatal examination.
2. Swellings in the pelvis are notoriously difficult to distinguish even by experts. The common causes are uterine fibroids, ovarian neoplastic cysts and inflammatory or endometriotic cysts. If there is any doubt, laparotomy should always be done because of the likelihood of ovarian cancer.
3. Non-menstrual, including postmenopausal, bleeding as a sign of uterine cancer is frequently neglected.
4. Early cancer of the cervix may be missed because of technical failure to expose the cervix to view.
5. Preinvasive carcinoma of the cervix may be missed because of failure to take a cytology smear accurately.
6. Vulval carcinoma may be overlooked in an elderly patient because itching, a common early symptom, may be treated without examination, sometimes for years.

In other words, overcome any inhibitions (often on the part of the patient) about vaginal examination, learn to expose the cervix with facility and to take a good cervical smear, and get specialist opinion on any swelling felt in the pelvis. Remember also that patients often visit their family doctor not expecting to be examined and therefore seem unwilling, but welcome an offer to return on another day after bathing.

Advanced Genital Cancer: Management and Cause of Death

Whatever the exact origin and type of genital cancers, they present the same clinical problems, which include:

1. Pain, especially due to invasion of bone.
2. Obstruction of bowel or ureters.
3. Bleeding ⎱
4. Infection ⎰ due to erosion through the vagina.
5. Urinary or faecal fistulae (connecting with the vagina) due to invasion of bladder or rectum.
6. Cachexia.

The commonest cause of death, in about half the cases, is uraemia resulting from ureteric obstruction – a relatively kind way. Cachexia, anaemia and infection account for most of the remainder.

The major problems to deal with are incontinence due to fistulae, which is demoralizing, and pain, which is dreaded. Radiotherapy may already be spent, and more irradiation may worsen the problem of ulceration by causing further necrosis of both tumour and normal tissue. Palliative surgery may be useful to divert faeces or urine by colostomy or ureteroileostomy, and if the tumour can be mobilized, exenteration (i.e. removal of rectum and/or bladder with the tumour) may be beneficial.

Pain is dreaded but need not be so. Doctors are frequently too inhibited in their use of analgesic drugs, partly because of their unwillingness to concede 'defeat' and accept a short-term outlook. Patients are usually more realistic than many doctors imagine, and can accept approaching death with calm and dignity given proper relief of their physical symptoms. When pain is unilateral, cord blockade using phenol may be effective, but, in general, oral analgesics are more appropriate. The important objective in treatment is to anticipate pain – it is much easier to keep it at bay than abolish it once established. The drugs should always be prescribed on a regular basis, not 'as required'. In this way mild analgesics, or pentazocine or methadone may suffice for a long time before morphine or heroin becomes necessary. Fears about narcotic addiction are out of place in these circumstances, and anyway the dose usually needs little increase once an effective level is reached and regularly maintained.

Other distressing symptoms include nausea, which can be relieved by phenothiazines, and anorexia, for which glucocorticoids may help by promoting normal anabolic metabolism which has been undermined by the tumour catabolism. Finally, there is no substitute for kind nursing.

Vulval Tumours

Benign Vulval Tumours
Dermal Tumours and Cysts
Sebaceous cysts, sweat gland tumours (hidradenomas), lipomas and fibromas occur on the labia majora as in skin elsewhere.

Bartholin's Cysts
This is a soft, unilocular cyst 2–5 cm in diameter, situated posterolaterally just outside the vaginal introitus. It represents the dilated duct of

Bartholin's gland, due to obstruction often by past infection, especially gonococcal. It is non-tender but may be a nuisance or worry. It may become secondarily infected resulting in a Bartholin's abscess. The best treatment is marsupialization, to restore permanent drainage. The ostium frequently closes again, however, especially when infected, and recurrence of the cyst is common.

Venereal Warts (Condylomata Acuminata)
These are viral in origin and may be venereally transmitted, being commonly associated with other venereal infections, notably that caused by *Trichomonas vaginalis*. They are cauliflower-like growths only a few millimetres in diameter, which may be isolated or may cluster over an extensive area. Treatment is by chemical cautery using podophyllin solution or, under anaesthesia, electrocautery or excision.

Syphilis
Syphilis may present as an ulcer on any part of the genital tract between the vulva and cervix, or as condylomata lata, which are moist, flat warts around the vulva. Condylomata lata may be associated with generalized lymphadenopathy and skin-rash, being manifestations of secondary syphilis. The lesions teem with *Treponema pallidum* which should be sought in scrapings by dark-ground microscopy. Genital ulcers and granulomata therefore need to be examined using protective gloves. For a more detailed account of syphilis *see* Chapter 3.

Urethral Prolapse, Caruncle and Carcinoma
A sliding prolapse of the posterior urethral mucosa often occurs, to a minor degree, in postmenopausal women and is due to lower urethral atrophy as a result of oestrogen deficiency. Physical exposure can then lead to the development of a granuloma, known as a urethral caruncle. This can cause dysuria and haematuria. It is usually easily recognized by its situation at the posterior margin of the external urinary meatus, but needs to be distinguished from urethral carcinoma and 'true' urethral prolapse.

'True' urethral prolapse means complete, annular eversion of the mucosa. It usually occurs due to oestrogen deficiency in elderly women, but occasionally in young girls. It may become strangulated and thus greatly swollen and haemorrhagic, and as a result can be confused with a malignant tumour of the vulva or vagina.

Urethral Cysts
See Vagina, *below*.

Vulval Dermatoses (Dystrophies)
Specific vulval dermatoses, or dystrophies, occur not uncommonly in middle and old age and always cause itching ('pruritis vulvae.). They must

be distinguished from general dermatoses, particularly psoriasis, which can affect the vulva as well as skin elsewhere. Some of the specific dermatoses are potentially malignant and can only be distinguished on biopsy. Diagnostic terminology is both confused and confusing. Common classification, with alternatives, is (a) kraurosis or senile atrophy, (b) lichen sclerosis et atrophicus, (c) leukoplakia or leukoplakic vulvitis. The following, however, is preferred.

Essentially, the lesion may be red because it is thin, or white because of a thick keratinized layer on the surface. It may also be excoriated and cracked due to scratching, but these same features may be due to early invasive carcinoma and should not go unsuspected. What matters is cellular activity and pleomorphism in the squamous epithelium, which must be determined histologically. And, because the degree of change varies in the whole field of the lesion, which may extend over most of the vulva, multiple biopsies are required. Histology may show:

atrophy
inflammation } 90 per cent of cases;

dysplasia
intraepithelial carcinoma } 10 per cent of cases.

Dysplasia and Intraepithelial Carcinoma

The distinction between the two is a matter of fine degree. Intraepithelial carcinoma is also called carcinoma in situ or Bowen's disease. The features are malignant change within the squamous cells, especially the nuclei, excess and abnormal mitotic figures, and lack of squamous differentiation in the epithelium, but an intact basal membrane.

These conditions occur in about one-third of cases in areas of chronic vulvitis (*see* Chapter 3) whatever the cause, including irritant chemicals and venereal granulomata (condylomata). The latter may be syphilitic, for which specific tests should be done, or viral, and, rarely, particularly in Negro immigrants to the UK, granuloma inguinale or lymphogranuloma venereum (*see* section on Venereal Diseases, Chapter 3).

Dysplasia and intraepithelial carcinoma are potentially invasive and must be treated, either by excision or by topical cytotoxic agent (5-fluorouracil). They are often extensive, and total vulvectomy may be required.

Benign Dermatoses

Atrophic or inflammatory dystrophies are occasionally due to diabetes mellitus and anaemia (of various causes), which should be sought. Otherwise treatment is symptomatic, the most effective agent being topical glucocorticoids. Oral antihistamines are useful at night for both antipruritic and sedative action. Vulvectomy is inappropriate because the skin drawn in to cover the area tends to undergo the original change.

Vulval Cancer
This is uncommon, accounting for 6 per cent of genital cancer, and in the UK occurs mainly in old age (Table 6.2). It is nearly always squamous. Basal cell, Bartholin's and urethral carcinoma, and sarcoma, are extremely rare.

Squamous carcinoma occurs as a proliferating or ulcerated lesion and presents because of its appearance or bleeding, but if neglected (as often occurs in old age) it may become infected. It spreads initially by local invasion and by lymphatic embolization to the superficial and deep inguinal nodes of both sides (*see Fig.* 2.8). Its aetiology is mainly unknown, but at least half – probably the majority – have been preceded by vulval dystrophy, which occurs on average about 10 years earlier and which in turn may often be due to chronic vulvitis.

Treatment at an early stage is by radical vulvectomy, i.e. total vulvectomy and regional lymphadenectomy. The extensive skin loss usually prevents primary wound healing, which largely occurs by granulation, thus requiring prolonged careful nursing. The resulting (corrected) 5-year survival is about 70 per cent, rising to 80 per cent in the absence of lymph node involvement, compared with about 50 per cent for all stages (Table 6.2). Radiotherapy is unsuitable because of the intense inflammatory response in the damaged, exposed tissue including surrounding dystrophic skin.

Vaginal Tumours

Benign Vaginal Tumours
Urethral Cysts
Urethral diverticulae and cysts of paraurethral glands, up to 4 cm diameter, occur in the lower anterior vaginal wall. If asymptomatic they are better left alone, because their removal may damage the urethra or lead to blockage of and cyst formation in the ducts of other paraurethral glands. If symptomatic they should not simply be incised; rather, expert help should be sought as their removal can be exceptionally difficult.

Dermal Inclusion Cysts
These usually occur in the lower posterior vaginal wall due to collected secretions from dermal tissue inadvertently buried when repairing a ragged laceration resulting from childbirth. They can be excised if a nuisance.

Mesonephric Duct Cysts
Also called Gartner's duct cysts, they occur in remnants of the mesonephric duct and thus occur in the anterolateral aspect of the upper vagina. They are about 5 cm in diameter, soft and not usually noticed by the patient. They are better left but can be excised if troublesome.

Vaginal Cancer
This is rare, accounting for less than 2 per cent of genital cancer. It is commonly secondary to cervical or endometrial carcinoma. Primary carcinoma of the vagina is usually squamous and occurs after the menopause, most commonly in association with ring pessary treatment of a prolapse. There has been, especially in the USA, a recent spate (although still rare) of adenocarcinoma in teenage girls following maternal treatment in early pregnancy (for threatened abortion) with stilboestrol – a fashion which has fortunately passed but should not be forgotten.

Vaginal carcinoma spreads into the paravaginal connective tissues, bladder and rectum, and by lymphatics both upwards to the cervical regional nodes and down to the vulval regional nodes (*see Fig.* 2.8). It is thus very difficult to treat radically, and the survival rate is low. Radiotherapy (intracavitary and beam) is usually most suitable.

Intraepithelial Squamous Carcinoma
Intraepithelial (preinvasive or in situ) squamous carcinoma may occur as a primary change in the vagina, but being invisible to the naked eye it is only recognized in practice when it occurs in association with known cervical squamous, usually preinvasive, carcinoma. It is then seen on colposcopy or exposed by its failure to stain with iodine (*see* Cervical Cancer, *below*).

It occurs in 4 per cent of cases of cervical intraepithelial squamous carcinoma. Although found as small isolated lesions these represent sporadic advances in what is a field change centred on the cervix. The lesions are thus usually found in the vaginal vault, sometimes after cervical conization or hysterectomy done for the cervical lesion, but may extend down to the vulva.

The lesions are potentially invasive and must be treated. Being often multiple, their local excision is impracticable (and some may be missed), and vaginectomy has been done in some cases. Now, however, the choice treatment is by topical cytotoxic therapy (using 5-fluorouracil), which seeks out all the neoplastic epithelium and causes only temporary inflammation of the normal.

Cervical Tumours

Benign Cervical Tumours
Mucous Polyp
This is a common pedunculated adenoma, up to 10 mm in diameter, arising from the endocervical mucosa and occurring at any age. It often bleeds, either on sexual intercourse, or spontaneously due to congestion or strangulation. If its pedicle can be seen and grasped the polyp can safely be twisted off when first seen at vaginal examination. The polyp may not be the cause of the bleeding, however, and after the menopause curettage is advisable to exclude endometrial carcinoma. Rarely, the polyp itself may be malignant.

Nabothian Follicles
These are mucous retention cysts, usually about 5 mm in diameter, beneath the squamous epithelium of the 'transitional zone' (*see below*) of the ectocervix. They have resulted from obstruction of gland-like mucosal crypts by squamous metaplasia in what was once surface mucosa. They are of no importance unless associated with chronic cervicitis (*see* Chapter 3), whilst in the taking of cervical smears they indicate the transitional zone.

Venereal Warts and Granulomata
Venereal warts (condylomata acuminata) may occur on the cervix (and less commonly in the vagina), as on the vulva (*see above*).

Granulomata, which sometimes bleed, may also occur on exposed endocervical mucosa when infected by *Trichomonas vaginalis*. They heal when the infection is eradicated.

Cervical Dystrophies and Preinvasive Carcinoma
Invasive squamous carcinoma of the cervix is invariably preceded by a preinvasive stage lasting some years. Every effort should be made to detect it at this stage when treatment is easy and effective. It usually arises in the epithelium close to the squamocolumnar junction (*see* Chapter 2). The epithelium here undergoes marked normal changes, but during particular phases it is specially susceptible to carcinogenic stimuli. It is therefore important to understand the normal changes that occur, as well as the dysplastic and neoplastic changes. These are all beautifully illustrated by Burghardt (1973).

Mucosal Ectopy, Squamous Metaplasia and the 'Transitional Zone'
The squamocolumnar junction is originally situated at the external cervical os. When the cervix grows under the stimulus of oestrogen, differential growth in the underlying parenchyma results in rolling out of the lips of the cervix and thus endocervical mucosa and the squamocolumnar junction are carried out onto the vaginal portion of the cervix. This effect is most marked in adolescence and first pregnancy. The exposure of the mucosa is called mucosal ectopy (or, wrongly, an 'erosion' because, being thin, it is bright red).

Physical exposure of the ectopic mucosa in the vagina leads to its metaplasia to squamous epithelium. This occurs initially by proliferation of 'reserve cells', i.e. normally isolated cells beneath the columnar epithelium. The proliferated reserve cells form stratified layers which then differentiate into normal squamous epithelium, and the columnar epithelium on the surface is eventually dislodged.

The underlying, gland-like mucosal crypts do not usually undergo squamous metaplasia but continue to secrete mucus via ostia in the surface squamous epithelium. They may become blocked, resulting in retention cysts (Nabothian follicles). These cysts, when they occur, provide the only clue visible to the naked eye of the area of previous mucosa that has undergone squamous metaplasia and called the 'transitional zone'. This zone is where squamous carcinoma invariably originates, because the cellular activity involved in the process of 'transition' seems to render the epithelium particularly susceptible to carcinogenic stimuli. It is therefore imperative that cancer cytology smears are taken from the area straddling the squamocolumnar junction and particularly just outside it, and wherever Nabothian follicles can be seen, which may be over an extensive area.

Dysplasia

Squamous epithelial dysplasia is characterized by basal hyperplasia (i.e. multi-layering of the basal cells), nuclear pleomorphism, and excessive and abnormal mitotic figures. When these changes occur mainly near the base of the squamous epithelium the condition is called 'mild dysplasia'. It usually resolves spontaneously and may, in some cases, be due to infection. When the changes extend close to the surface of the epithelium the condition is called 'severe dysplasia'. This is very unlikely to revert to normal, but will eventually proceed to invasive carcinoma in most cases. Severe dysplasia is therefore a form of (differentiated) intraepithelial carcinoma and should be treated accordingly (*see* Carcinoma in situ, *below*).

The distinction between mild and severe dysplasia is thus of great clinical importance but, being a matter of degree only, can be difficult to make. A third category, 'moderate dysplasia', is sometimes used to indicate doubt.

The individual cytological appearances (i.e. in a smear) associated with dysplasia (which is a histological diagnosis) are typically dyskaryosis. This means pleomorphic (i.e. malignant-looking) nuclei set in otherwise normally differentiated (i.e. expanded, typically squamous) cytoplasm.

Carcinoma in situ

This is characterized by nuclear pleomorphism and excessive and abnormal mitotic figures at all levels in the squamous epithelium with lack of any squamous differentiation throughout the thickness of the epithelium. It represents a form of intraepithelial squamous carcinoma which is undifferentiated, in contrast to 'severe dysplasia', which is differentiated.

Carcinoma in situ was originally defined as described because its appearances were indisputable, unlike severe and mild dysplasia. This expediency has unfortunately led to confusion about the relative clinical implications of carcinoma in situ and severe dysplasia – these should be considered as the same, being different only in their degrees of differentiation (*see* Table 6.3).

The risk of intraepithelial carcinoma becoming invasive is high, and spontaneous resolution is very unlikely. There remains some uncertainty about the exact risk, because biopsy for histological diagnosis is likely to interfere excessively (if not completely) with the lesion and its natural

Table 6.3.   Summary of cervical epithelial dystrophies and neoplasia related to their clinical implications and required treatment

Lesion		Treatment
Reserve cell hyperplasia ⎫ normal		Disregard
Squamous metaplasia ⎭		
Mild dysplasia		Observe
Severe dysplasia ⎫ intraepithelial ⎫		Local
Carcinoma in situ ⎬ carcinoma ⎬		excision-biopsy
Microinvasive carcinoma ⎭		
Invasive carcinoma		Extended or radical surgery/radiotherapy

development. Nevertheless, it seems clear that invasion will probably occur in nearly all cases eventually, the average time-lag being about 10 years. This means that treatment by local excision is adequate and, although desirable, there is no immediate urgency for it (thus it can be postponed in pregnancy, for instance).

Microinvasive Carcinoma
This is characterized by loss of integrity of the basal membrane, at least in parts, of otherwise intraepithelial carcinoma with microscopic carcinomatous invasion of the underlying stroma to a maximum depth of 5 mm. (Unfortunately, different criteria of depth have been used in various studies, but 5 mm is commonly used in current practice.) By international convention it is called stage 1a(i) squamous carcinoma (*see* Table 6.4), but it can be treated conservatively as for intraepithelial carcinoma (which is called stage 0). Table 6.3 shows more clearly the practical divisions between the cervical epithelial dystrophies and carcinoma.

The safety of conservative treatment is sometimes still doubted – and hysterectomy may be preferred in older women with complete families – although proven. The safety margin is emphasized by the virtually total survival rate associated also with early ('occult') invasive carcinoma (stage 1a(ii): *see* Table 6.4). Although that is treated radically the results imply that embolic spread does not occur until the invasive tumour has progressed a further step in size (to stage 1b: *see* Table 6.4). In this respect total tumour volume is probably more important then depth of invasion alone, and 0·5 cm³ might be a better limit for the definition of microinvasive carcinoma. *See below* for details of treatment.

Diagnosis and Treatment of Preinvasive Carcinoma
Naked Eye Examination
Preinvasive (including microinvasive) carcinoma is invisible to the naked

eye. Naked eye examination is, however, an essential part of 'screening' for cervical carcinoma to detect an invasive lesion, because cytology is much more likely to produce a false negative result with invasive than with preinvasive carcinoma (due to surface necrosis). For this reason (amongst others) there is no place for 'blind' cytology, using aspirate from the vaginal vault, in the diagnosis of cervical lesions.

Cytology

The accessibility and small target area make the cervix very suitable for cytological examination. This is best done on a smear made from fresh cells scraped directly from the surface of the cervix (Ayre's smear), in

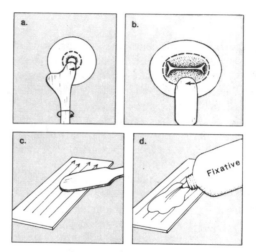

Fig. 6.2. How to take a good cervical smear. (The shaded area on the cervix represents mucosa.) *a* and *b*, Taking the scrape from around the squamocolumnar junction of a nulliparous cervix with little mucosa visible, or a parous cervix with moderate mucosal ectopy. *c*, Spreading the smear to achieve a series of thin wedges. *d*, Immediate fixing while the cells are fresh.

contrast to true exfoliative cytology of posterior fornix aspirate (Papanicolaou smear). The latter sometimes affords detection of endometrial and rarely ovarian carcinoma but is not wholly reliable for those purposes. It is preferable to concentrate attention on the cervix, best done using the scrape smear. This must be taken accurately, from the area of the squamocolumnar junction and surrounding transitional zone (*see above*), as demonstrated in *Fig.* 6.2. The smear must be spread so as to achieve ample areas only one cell thick for proper microscopical examination, and must be fixed in a fresh state, as shown.

To check that the smear has been taken from the right areas on the cervix both squamous and columnar cells should be present (and reported) in ample proportions. Malignant and/or dyskaryotic cells are sought, but these are sometimes reported in terms, already interpreted, of the expected histological findings ('mild or severe dysplasia, carcinoma in situ'). Incidental findings that are sometimes useful include cellular inflammatory changes, sometimes specifically recognizable as due to herpes or cytomegalovirus; monilial strands and *Trichomonas vaginalis*; and changes indicating oestrogen state.

Cervical cancer cytology may be used to screen healthy women or as a test of cure following local treatment of preinvasive carcinoma. The pick-up rate of cytological neoplasia is about 5 per 1000 smears but depends on age and whether the population has been screened before and how often. It is much higher in certain groups of women, for instance those in prison or attending venereology clinics. False positive findings occur rarely and anyway are unimportant. They are usually not false, being explained by technical error in taking the (negative) biopsy, and should be pursued by repeated cytology. The finding of malignant cells in a smear can never be disregarded. False negatives are of great concern. They occur in about 10 per cent of new cases, the majority being due to observer error which is to be expected when screening. In following up known cases the error occurs in only about 3 per cent. These may be due to inaccurate collection or improper preparation of the smear. A negative smear is sometimes found shortly after a positive one – which is then wrongly assumed to have been false – because much of the abnormal epithelium may have been scraped off at the original test. A smear should therefore not be repeated in less than a month.

In planning cytological screening schedules the false negative rate must be taken into account as well as the natural history of intraepithelial carcinoma. Repeating the first smear after a year will reduce the false negative rate to about 1 per cent, which seems acceptable, and thereafter smears every 3–5 years should not overlook any cases prior to invasion.

It remains questionable whether cytological screening actually reduces deaths from cervical cancer. It has been argued that some invasive carcinomas occur with little or no preinvasive stage and are therefore always likely to be missed, but this is improbable. What is true is that the incidence of cervical carcinoma is gradually falling everywhere, unrelated to cytology screening, probably due to improved socioeconomic conditions. However, the long natural history of preinvasive carcinoma, and further survival after invasive carcinoma has been treated, will require a delay of about 20 years before any effect of cytology screening on cervical cancer mortality might be seen. Unfortunately, women most at risk tend to use the service least. Amongst screened women the incidence of invasive cervical carcinoma has undoubtedly been reduced by treatment of preinvasive carcinoma. The more worrying question, at least in the UK, is the financial disincentive to screen women under 35 years old. Increasing teenage coitus and pregnancy (*see* Aetiology, *below*) is leading to a steady rise in cervical cancer in women in their twenties.

Colposcopy

The colposcope is a binocular instrument that allows X 5–10 magnification of the cervix. It is positioned outside the vagina, making it easy to use, and the view is obtained with the help of an ordinary vaginal speculum.

The colposcope cannot be used to detect cytological detail within the epithelium nor invasion from the basal layers. Its usefulness depends on the pattern of the vascular supply that is so closely related to the degree of epithelial neoplasia. The vessels are larger and are carried (in loops) closer to the surface than normal between the rete pegs, giving rise to an appearance of punctation on the surface. In more advanced lesions the punctation occurs in close alignments giving rise to mosaic patterns. Branching vessels running on the surface suggest invasive carcinoma. (For illustration *see* Langley, 1976.)

Colposcopy is relatively time-consuming and therefore not practicable for screening. It is used as an adjunct to cytology once neoplastic cells have been found. It has two major applications:

1. To define the extent of intraepithelial carcinoma so that surgical excision can be minimized. Tiny lesions can be excised by punch biopsy without anaesthesia. If cone biopsy is required its dimensions can be prescribed for the surgeon. (Before colposcopy was available very large cones were taken, resulting in unfortunate damage risking future fertility — *see below*.)
2. To observe mild dysplasia (usually associated with mild dyskaryosis on cytology) without treatment until either it regresses or advances to severe dysplasia needing excision. Observation by colposcopy needs to be repeated every 6–12 months.

Non-specific Staining

Iodine. Normal cervical squamous epithelium, whether original or metaplastic, contains glycogen which is stained by iodine, unlike dysplastic squamous epithelium. Lack of staining does not give any clue to the severity of the lesion, but it provides the surgeon with excellent definition of the area to be excised for cone biopsy.

Acetic Acid. This gives dysplastic squamous epithelium an opaque appearance. It is therefore sometimes used at colposcopy, especially as it removes mucus, but it tends to obscure the vascular pattern.

Treatment

Intraepithelial carcinoma (severe dysplasia or carcinoma in situ) and microinvasive carcinoma should be treated by local excision (*see* Table

6.3). Ablation by cautery, or possibly in the future by laser, is also effective, but excision biopsy is better in order to confirm the cytological and colposcopic diagnosis and to definitely exclude invasion. When the lesion is extensive, cone biopsy is necessary, the limits of the biopsy being prescribed by colposcopy and/or iodine staining. Because the severity of the lesion varies in its different parts, histological examination needs to be comprehensive: 10–20 sections are taken from all parts. If the lesion is seen not to be completely excised in the cone, re-conization can be done.

The immediate risks of cone biopsy are haemorrhage and infection, particularly because the bed of the cone is best left exposed to re-epithelialize (from its edges and from the remaining depths of divided crypts). This is done so that any lesion remaining in the crypts will be exposed for subsequent cytology, this being the test of cure.

Cone biopsy also involves particular risks to future fertility, by excessive loss of mucus-secreting crypts (which are mainly situated in the lower part of the cervix), and by incompetence of the internal os in pregnancy. Oddly enough stenosis of the cervical canal can also be a sequel.

Hysterectomy is sometimes chosen, out of super-caution, as treatment in older women who have completed their families, especially when there is microinvasion. This does not remove the need, however, to maintain indefinite annual cytological follow-up on the remaining nearby tissues, including the vaginal vault, which continue to be at particular risk.

Cervical Cancer

Invasive tumours of the cervix may be:

squamous cell carcinoma (95 per cent);
adenocarcinoma (5 per cent);
sarcoma (very rare, usually botryoid (i.e. grape-like) sarcoma in children).

They mostly occur on the ectocervix and are usually exophytic or ulcerative, giving rise to bleeding, typically on coitus. Endocervical carcinoma (usually adenocarcinoma) tends to be mainly infiltrative and may expand the cervix without broaching the surface of the ectocervix, which, however, becomes irregular, firm and vascular. In this case bleeding also occurs but not so readily on coitus.

As *Fig.* 6.1 shows, the incidence of cervical cancer is high from the age of 40 years onwards, and not uncommon from 30 to 39 years. Indeed the incidence in younger women has been steadily increasing, so that cervical cancer is now not rare even in women aged 20–29 years. This change reflects changes in social and sexual behaviour concerned with the aetiology of squamous cell carcinoma.

Aetiology

The outstanding aetiological factors in squamous carcinoma of the cervix are coitus and early age of coitus. The actual carcinogenic agent seems most likely to be sperm DNA. Herpesvirus type 2 was, at one time, a hot favourite but now seems less likely a cause.

Cervical cancer is extremely rare in virgins, shown for instance by studies in nuns. Youth is important probably because this is when squamous metaplasia in ectopic mucosa is most active and thus the epithelium most susceptible to carcinogenesis. All other demonstrable aetiological associations are probably related to early coitus: low socioeconomic status, early marriage, high parity, promiscuity, prostitution and venereal disease. Ritual male circumcision was once thought to be protective, as in Jews and Moslems, but the relatively low incidence of cervical cancer in these groups is probably related to cultural differences affecting coital behaviour.

Treatment and Prognosis
The mode of treatment depends on the way in which the cancer spreads and on the extent of spread (Table 6.4). Cervical cancer spreads initially

Table 6.4. Clinical staging of cervical squamous carcinoma, required treatment and resulting success

Clinical stage		Treatment	5-year survival rate (corrected) %
0.	Intraepithelial	Local excision-biopsy	100
1a (i).	Microinvasive		
1a (ii).	Occult (symptomless) invasive		100
1b.	Overt, limited to cervix	Radical radiotherapy or surgery	80
2.	Involving upper vagina and/or parametrium not as far as pelvic side walls		60
3.	Extending to pelvic side walls and/or lower vagina	Radical radiotherapy	30
4.	Extending to bladder, rectum or outside true pelvis	Palliative radiotherapy and/or pelvic exenteration	10

by local invasion (to the vaginal vault and/or parametrium) and to lymph nodes within the pelvis (internal and external iliac, and obturator, nodes: see Fig. 2.8). Thus in its early stages it lends itself to radical therapy, i.e. aimed at the tumour and the pelvic lymphatic field. Radiotherapy is now generally preferred to radical (Wertheim) hysterectomy because radiotherapeutic skills can be better developed by concentration in large centres. Intracavitary irradiation (i.e. using sources placed in the cervical canal, vaginal vault and uterine cavity) is usually combined with external beam therapy to the lateral lymphatic fields. More advanced cancer is usually treated by beam therapy to the whole pelvis, but palliative surgery is occasionally appropriate (see Advanced Genital Cancer, above).

The prognosis depends on the stage reached by the tumour before treatment (Table 6.4). The staging is of course done clinically, and the failure of treatment in some cases at stages 1 and 2 is due to the presence already of clinically undetectable embolization beyond the pelvic lymph nodes. Although the 5-year survival rate of overt stage 1 cervical cancer is 80 per cent, the majority of cases of cervical cancer present much later, resulting in less than half of the patients surviving overall (Table 6.2). These poor results are tragic because they would mostly be avoidable if prompt attention were paid to the bleeding that invariably occurs at an early stage.

Tumours of the Uterine Body

Gross enlargement of the uterus is usually due to benign myometrial tumours ('fibroids') and may or may not be associated with symptoms (usually menorrhagia). Modest enlargement is commonly due to overall hypertrophy associated with premenopausal anovulatory cycles and menorrhagia; or it may be due to endometrial carcinoma. Endometrial carcinoma, however, usually presents at an early stage with bleeding, before any uterine enlargement has occurred.

Benign Tumours
'Fibroids'

Fibroids are the commonest uterine tumours. They are leiomyomas, sometimes called fibromyomas, arising in the myometrium. They are firm, round, well defined tumours with a whorled pattern on the cut surface. They are usually multiple; sometimes there appears to be one alone but close examination usually reveals many other small ones. They are benign and rarely progress to sarcoma. Their origin is uncertain but may be from vascular elements. They are particularly likely to occur in Negro women and in women remaining nulliparous after the age of 30 years. Fibroids are clearly dependent on ovarian hormones because they occur in the reproductive epoch, grow particularly in pregnancy and regress after the menopause. They may outgrow their vascular supply in pregnancy and undergo infarction with internal bleeding ('acute or red degeneration'). After the menopause gradual, hyaline degeneration occurs.

Fibroids cause symptoms as a result of:

1. Their exact situation in the uterus (*Fig. 6.3*);
2. Acute accidents to them;
3. Their size.

Very large subserous fibroids causing abdominal swelling may otherwise be symptomless. However, fibroids that enlarge or distort the uterine cavity cause painless menorrhagia – the most characteristic feature. Submucous fibroids may interfere with implantation of the blastocyst, causing infertility. Pedunculated submucous fibroids may be extruded through the

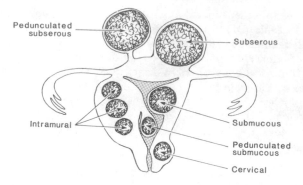

Fig. 6.3. Fibroids – their various situations in the uterus (the related significance described in the text).

cervix and become strangulated causing severe bleeding. Pedunculated subserous fibroids may undergo torsion causing severe pain. Acute (red) degeneration in pregnancy causes severe pain which tempts surgical exploration but will resolve in a few days if treated conservatively. Fibroids situated in the cervix obstruct labour but are fortunately rare.

A rare and unexplained association with fibroids is polycythaemia, which in some cases disappears after hysterectomy.

Fibroids need to be removed only if they cause symptoms, although large fibroids are sometimes removed only for fear of the tiny risk of sarcoma. Hysterectomy is the usual choice. Myomectomy (i.e. ennucleation of the fibroids from the uterus, which is conserved) is done only to preserve fertility because it is usually a more difficult operation, involving the removal of many fibroids, and because it is more dangerous on account of bleeding and associated greater postoperative morbidity.

Adenomyoma/Adenomyosis
These represent the fibromyomatous reaction to internal endometriosis, i.e. endometrial tissue situated deep in the myometrium and continuous with the normal endometrium. It leads to enlargement of the uterus. The condition may be diffuse (adenomyosis) or localized (adenomyoma). It causes menorrhagia but, unlike a fibroid, an adenomyoma causes pain and is poorly circumscribed. For the latter reason hysterectomy is the only means of treatment.

Connective Tissue and Vascular Tumours of the Myometrium
Fibromas, lymphangiomas, haemangiomas and haemangiopericytomas are rare. However, it has been postulated that fibroids may originate as haemangiopericytomas.

Uterine Hypertrophy
Generalized enlargement of the uterus, two or threefold, sometimes occurs in association with menorrhagia in the last menstrual decade. It is probably due to the effect of oestrogen unopposed by any progesterone, associated with anovulatory cycles. The menorrhagia should be treated as 'dysfunctional bleeding' (*see* Chapter 5) by the use of hormones, despite the uterine size.

Endometrial Adenoma ('Benign Polyp')
This is a soft, red, fleshy tumour of the endometrium, which may be sessile or pedunculated, and is prone to bleed irregularly. If pedunculated it may appear through the cervix, and may then become strangulated and bleed profusely. It varies in size from about 1 cm diameter, if it consists only of endometrium, up to 5 cm, if it includes a myometrial or fibrous framework.

The diagnosis is made by curettage which is done because of irregular bleeding, and the procedure is curative. Paradoxically, it may seem, the larger polyps are more likely to be missed at curettage and are usually discovered at hysterectomy done for intractable bleeding.

Not all endometrial polyps are benign; histological examination must always be made.

Endometrial Hyperplasia
There are two different types, one benign and the other with high malignant potential. They both tend to occur in the last menstrual decade.

Cystic Hyperplasia
This results from prolonged oestrogen stimulation unopposed by any progesterone, i.e. anovulatory menstrual cycles. The cycles are often prolonged and associated with heavy menstrual bleeding, and this syndrome is called 'metropathia haemorrhagica'. The endometrium is thickened and often polypoid. Both the glands and stroma show mitotic activity and many of the glands are markedly dilated. On section the distended glands are visible to the naked eye, giving rise to the description of 'Swiss cheese appearance'.

Cystic hyperplasia affects the whole endometrium. It is a benign condition of no danger and is responsive to progesterone, which when withdrawn results in normal shedding of the endometrium.

Adenomatous ('Atypical') Hyperplasia
This is a focal condition involving only the glands, which become crowded together. It varies in degree. When there is intraluminal folding and tufting of the glandular epithelium with cellular pleomorphism it is sometimes called 'carcinoma in situ'. It causes bleeding.

Adenomatous hyperplasia depends on oestrogen but, unlike cystic hyperplasia, does not seem to depend on excessive oestrogen and is only partly responsive to progesterone. The risk of progression to invasive carcinoma is about 20 per cent so treatment is mandatory. Curettage may be effective but must be repeated. Hysterectomy is the usual choice because the lesion generally occurs after the age of 40 years in women who have completed their families.

Cancer of the Uterine Body
Invasive tumours originating in the body of the uterus include:

Endometrial
    adenocarcinoma
    squamous cell carcinoma
    stromal sarcoma
Myometrial
    leiomyosarcoma
Trophoblastic (conceptual)
    hydatidiform mole (invasive type)
    choriocarcinoma.

In practice nearly all are endometrial adenocarcinoma. Of the others, the invasive trophoblastic tumours are the most important because they are often curable (in the true sense). Delay in diagnosis of choriocarcinoma is particularly tragic because it is often a young mother who will die, and that could have been avoided.

Endometrial adenocarcinoma
This may involve the endometrium generally, or focally in the form of a polyp or polyps. Histologically there are usually glandular ('tubular') formations typical of endometrium. Invasion of the myometrium occurs to a variable extent, and some bulky tumours expanding the uterus three or fourfold may invade very little. The tumour is soft and friable, and vaginal bleeding usually occurs at an early stage so that most cases come to light while the uterus is still normal in size and the walls unbroached. Occasionally, tumour obstructs the cervical canal, leading to a painful pyometra (pus-filled uterus).

    Endometrial adenocarcinoma occurs most often in the two decades after the menopause and is rare before it (*see Fig.* 6.1 and Table 6.2). In contrast to cervical squamous cell carcinoma, it is increasing in incidence and is relatively more common in the higher socioeconomic classes. The associated features classically described, of obesity, hypertension, nulliparity and often diabetes mellitus, are open to question. The only clear association is with oestrogen but it does not seem to depend on the amount. The particular oestrogen is possibly the important factor, e.g. oestrone which is relatively predominant after the menopause as a result of extraglandular conversion (in subcutaneous fat) from adrenocortical precursors. Endometrial cancer is occasionally due to an oestrogen-secreting ovarian tumour, usually a granulosa cell tumour. Progestogens probably protect against endometrial cancer by their antioestrogenic action, and their cyclical inclusion in postmenopausal oestrogen therapy seems to be an important safeguard.

Adenomatous hyperplasia is a common but not invariable precursor of endometrial cancer. Screening for and treating adenomatous hyperplasia would unfortunately not offer a reliable means of preventing endometrial carcinoma.

Endometrial cancer spreads initially by lymphatics and involves the para-aortic nodes directly via the ovarian vascular route (see Fig. 2.8), by seeding to the ovary (through the Fallopian tube) in about 10 per cent of cases and to the vagina (through the cervix), and later by embolization in the blood. The tumour tends to be confined to the uterus and does not break through its walls until a late stage. The depth of invasion of the myometrium correlates well with lymph node involvement and provides the best prognostic index.

Primary lymphatic spread beyond the pelvis makes radical therapy (as applied to cervical carcinoma) inappropriate. Endometrial adenocarcinoma is also less sensitive to radiotherapy than cervical squamous cell carcinoma. Treatment (Table 6.5) is thus primarily by hysterectomy and bilateral

Table 6.5. **Clinical staging of endometrial carcinoma, required treatment and resulting success**

Stage	Treatment	5-year survival rate (corrected) %
1. Confined to uterine body	Surgery with local radiotherapy	90
2. Involves cervix	Surgery with irradiation of whole pelvis	50
3. Extending outside uterus but confined to pelvis	Irradiation of whole pelvis with surgery if possible	25
4. Extending outside pelvis or including bladder or rectum	As for stage 3, plus irradiation of isolated metastases or progestogen therapy	5

salpingo-oophorectomy. More extensive resection is sometimes done, particularly including removal of the upper vagina, but is of no proven benefit. Additional radiotherapy aimed at the uterus and upper vagina reduces the risk of pelvic recurrence of tumour after operation. It may be given postoperatively to destroy any seeds disseminated by operative manipulation, or preoperatively to inhibit tumour activity and so prevent any operative seeding. Pre- and postoperative irradiation seems equally effective. More extensive radiotherapy may be appropriate in more advanced cases, to the regional lymph nodes and isolated distant metastases. Extensive metastasis can be checked in about a third of cases, and complete regression occasionally achieved, by progestogen therapy in prolonged high dosage. Progestogen therapy while the tumour is confined to the uterus does not seem to improve on the good results of hysterectomy and local radiotherapy (Table 6.5). In general the survival rate with endometrial carcinoma is good (see Table 6.2) because most cases present relatively early, the tumour being slow to spread beyond the uterus.

Trophoblastic Tumours and 'Trophoblast Disease'
The tumours arising from trophoblast are the hydatidiform mole and choriocarcinoma, described below. Choriocarcinomas are mostly highly malignant, whereas hydatidiform moles are mostly benign. The invasive potential and vigour of any individual tumour cannot, however, be distinguished histologically. Normal trophoblast also has the capacity to invade and spread – it is often found deep in the myometrium, and emboli reaching the lungs occasionally cause haemoptysis – but it does not persist. The concept has thus developed of 'trophoblast disease', i.e. a spectrum of trophoblastic invasiveness and neoplasia ranging from the normal to cancers of extreme malignancy, and whose activity (and size) is best determined by HCG production, which is indicated by levels in blood or urine. Trophoblast disease thus includes:

metastatic normal trophoblast
hydatidiform mole (1 in 2000 pregnancies)
    benign (90 per cent)
    malignant ('invasive mole')
choriocarcinoma (1 in 20 000 pregnancies).

AETIOLOGY
Trophoblastic tumours occur much more commonly in Chinese Asians and more commonly in Negro women than in Europeans. The tumour karyotype appears to be female in most cases. This is possibly due to multiple fertilization of the oocyte or to spermatozoal abnormalities characterized by extra X chromosomes, the latter being suggested by occasional examples of trophoblast tumours occurring in numerous consecutive pregnancies.

HYDATIDIFORM MOLE
This occurs in about 1 in 2000 pregnancies amongst European women. The tumour consists of distended fluid-filled chorionic villi lacking fetal blood vessels. It forms a grape-like mass of vesicles each 3–5 mm in diameter. It involves the whole chorion and there is no fetus. The absence of the fetus results inevitably in abortion, and other clinical features

depend on the sometimes excessive mass of the tumour (in relation to the gestational age) and the excessive production of HCG. Thus it usually presents like a threatened abortion and with one or more of the following features:

vaginal bleeding;
excessive vomiting;
hypertension (pre-eclampsia);
excessive uterine size;
doughy uterine consistency (instead of cystic).

The differential diagnoses are multiple pregnancy and acute polyhydramnios. The diagnostic features are the absent fetal heart, the sonogram which shows the multiple echoes from the vesicles looking like a snowstorm, and abnormally high levels of HCG. An occasional feature is ovarian enlargement by theca-lutein cysts due to excess HCG.

Treatment is by suction evacuation of the uterus (as for vaginal termination of pregnancy). This is better than curettage or induction of abortion using oxytocic agents because these methods increase the likelihood of embolization of the tumour. Usually some tumour, having invaded the myometrium, persists for a while, but spontaneous regression occurs in 90 per cent of cases within 6 months. Until then, the tumour need not be treated so long as HCG levels are declining. These levels need to be measured every 2 weeks at first. HCG provides the test of cure but should remain undetectable for 2 years before the risk of resurgent growth from persisting microscopic invasive tumours can confidently be eliminated. Meanwhile a further pregnancy would cause dangerous confusion and should be avoided. Oral contraceptives delay regression of the tumour and their use should be postponed until HCG is undetectable.

Persistence, progression or metastasis (indicating malignancy: 'invasive mole') occur in 5 per cent of cases and need to be treated as for choriocarcinoma. A further 5 per cent give rise to actual choriocarcinoma.

CHORIOCARCINOMA
This occurs in about 1 in 20 000 pregnancies, about half following hydatidiform mole and the other half following equally abortion or childbirth. Very rarely choriocarcinoma may originate in the ovary (as in the testicle). The tumour consists of sheets of syncytio- and cytotrophoblast without villi. It is soft, highly vascular and bleeds readily; indeed death from choriocarcinoma is most commonly due to bleeding, either at the original site in the pelvis, or from pulmonary or sometimes cerebral metastases.

The presenting symptom is usually vaginal bleeding. Although this often follows a known hydatidiform mole it also often occurs some weeks or months after unremarkable childbirth or abortion. Persistent or irregular bleeding after childbirth or abortion should therefore never be ignored (although much more likely to be due to ordinary retained placental tissue). The diagnosis is made by curettage.

Treatment is by intermittent chemotherapy using combinations of cytotoxic agents. The tumour response is monitored by means of HCG levels. The high risk of granulocytopenia and consequent infection can be reduced by isolation of the patient in a sterilized 'cell'. Large pelvic tumours may require surgical excision; otherwise complete remission with preservation of normal reproductive function can be expected in 75 per cent of cases. If the tumour is detected early nearly all patients should be cured.

Tumours of the Fallopian Tube

These are extremely rare. Various benign tumours of connective tissue can occur. Malignant tumours (usually adenocarcinoma) represent much less than 1 per cent of genital cancer. They occur after the menopause and present with vaginal bleeding or sanguinous or even watery discharge and/or pelvic mass, and are usually only diagnosed at laparotomy. Spread outside the tube has usually already occurred, and despite surgery and/or radiotherapy the survival rate is poor.

Ovarian Tumours

The symptoms of ovarian tumours and in some cases the mode of treatment are determined by the histological type and whether benign or malignant. The tumours will therefore be considered under these headings.

Histopathological Classification of Ovarian Tumours

There is a very great variety of ovarian tumours as shown in Table 6.6. Disordered follicular growth resulting in cysts occurs of course only in premenopausal women and accounts for about half the ovarian tumours in young women. Endometriotic cysts also occur only before the menopause, being dependent on oestrogen, but are uncommon. Of the neoplastic tumours occurring in young women, dermoid cysts and sex-cord tumours are relatively common, although the epithelial (serous and mucinous) cysts are commonest at all ages.

Table 6.7 shows that of ovarian neoplasms 80 per cent are cystic (serous, mucinous or dermoid). As serous or mucinous cysts become malignant the proliferative parts contribute greater solidity to the tumour, while malignant teratomata (the malignant counterpart of dermoid cysts, which are benign teratomata) are almost entirely solid. About 20 per cent of ovarian neoplasms are solid and of these the majority are malignant. Many solid tumours secrete sex steroids (the sex-cord tumours).

Follicular Cysts

These are derived from ovarian follicles. The normal Graafian follicle reaches up to 1·5 cm diameter. Further enlargement up to 5 cm is called a

Table 6.6.   Classification of the majority of ovarian tumours

Origin and type	Benign (B) Malignant (M) Low-grade malignancy (LM)	Remarks
NON-NEOPLASTIC		
1. Follicular		Common, premenopausal
non-luteinized follicular cyst		
corpus luteum cyst		
theca-lutein cysts		
2. Endometriotic		
NEOPLASTIC		
1. Epithelial (i.e. from coelomic		
epithelium)		
serous cyst	B or M	common
mucinous cyst	B or M	common
endometrioid carcinoma	M	
Brenner tumour	B	
2. Sex-cord tumours (i.e. from		
cortical mesenchyme)		
granulosa cell tumour	LM	usually oestrogenic, thecoma-
theca cell tumour (usually	B	fibroma fairly common
thecoma-fibroma)		
tubular androblastoma	LM	
(arrhenoblastoma)		usually androgenic
hilus cell (Leydig cell) tumour	LM	
gynandroblastoma	LM	mixed steroidogenic
3. Germ cell tumours (i.e. from pri-		
mordial germ cells or oocytes)		
teratoma (benign form =	B or M	embryonic cell types;
'dermoid' cyst)		'dermoid' cyst common
endodermal sinus tumour	M	
(secretes AFP)		extraembryonic cell types
choriocarcinoma (secretes	M	
HCG)		
dysgerminoma	M	undifferentiated
4. Connective tissue tumours		
fibroma	B or M	
lipoma		
5. Metastatic tumour	all M	
commonly gastrointestinal		

AFP = alphafetoprotein.
HCG = human chorionic gonadotrophin.

'cystic follicle' and can be ignored. Enlargement greater than 5 cm is more likely to be due to a neoplastic cyst and can never be ignored (see Treatment of Ovarian Cysts, below). Their very presence implies disordered ovarian function and they are often associated with menstrual disturbance. However, they may also be symptomless, or only cause symptoms suddenly, due to an accidental complication (see Complications of Benign Ovarian Tumours, below).

Table 6.7.   The proportionate (percentage) incidence of ovarian neoplasms by cystic or solid state, by individual cystic types and by benign or malignant state

Type of Neoplasm	Benign	Malignant	Total
Serous Cysts	26	7	33
Mucinous Cysts	23	6	29
Dermoid Cysts	18	–	18
Total Cysts	67	13	80
Solid Tumours	8	12	20
Totals	75	25	100

Corpus luteum cysts arise as a result of haemorrhage (the blood usually later having been resorbed) into a previously normal corpus luteum. The prominent luteinized granulosa cell layer is characteristic, and these cysts occur singly.

Theca-lutein cysts are uncommon, being associated with trophoblast tumours and due to the high levels of HCG. They are multiple and the theca is prominently luteinized, in contrast to the normal corpus luteum.

Endometriotic Cysts

These are uncommon. They are always filled with blood, partly altered, due to regular menstruation – hence representing the typical (but not the only) example of so-called chocolate cysts. Being surrounded by inflammatory reaction they cause pain and fixation as well as swelling of the ovary (*see* Chapter 3).

Epithelial Cysts

These are thought to be derived from the coelomic epithelium of the ovary. Remembering the close embryonic relations of the various structures of the genitourinary tract (*see* Chapter 2), it is not surprising that the ovarian epithelial tumours bear histological resemblance to the normal epithelia of the Fallopian tube (serous cysts), endometrium (endometrioid carcinoma), endocervical mucosa (mucinous cysts) and urinary tract (Brenner tumours).

Serous cysts are usually unilocular and mucinous cysts often multilocular. They are usually thin-walled, lined by the active epithelium and surrounded by a smooth fibrous capsule. Epithelial secretions form the cyst and lead to its enlargement. Some reach football size. Malignant proliferation first leads to heaping up of the epithelium within the cyst; at this stage cystectomy is usually curative. Later, the capsule is invaded and tumour excrescences appear on the outer surface of the cyst, and the general tumour structure becomes semi-solid. About a quarter of epithelial cysts are malignant or are likely to progress to malignancy. Epithelial carcinomas of the ovary are bilateral in about 20 per cent of cases, often due to metastasis but sometimes originally. Benign tumours are occasionally bilateral; therefore, in practice, when a cyst is found the other ovary should be carefully examined and, if the patient is over 40, removed together with the uterus.

Endometrioid tumours are always malignant and solid. They need to be distinguished from metastatic endometrial carcinoma. Thus when a solid ovarian tumour is found diagnostic curettage is mandatory.

Brenner tumours (named after the man who first described them) are hard tumours, being composed of tiny islands of transitional or squamous epithelium set in a dense fibrous stroma. They are uncommon and benign.

Sex-Cord Tumours

Sex-cord tumours are so called because in the embryonic differentiation of granulosa and theca cells from the ovarian cortex (*see* Chapter 1) the cortex first differentiates into radial cords (the 'sex cords'), which later break up into the typical follicular arrangements. The sex cords also involve the primordial medulla, which, although it mostly regresses in the ovary, gives rise to the androgen-secreting hilus cells; these are analogous with the testicular Leydig (interstitial) cells.

The histological variants of sex-cord tumours shown in Table 6.6 should thus be self-evident. These tumours secrete sex hormones which are usually typical of their cell type. The presenting features of these tumours are usually due to their hormone secretion: menstrual disturbances, postmenopausal bleeding associated with proliferative endometrium or virilization. When a tumour is suspected in these circumstances the ovary may need to be visualized by laparoscopy or even split open at laparotomy because these tumours may be very small (although they vary greatly in size). They are solid and unilateral.

The majority of sex-cord tumours are malignant but not very aggressive, being mainly only locally invasive. The commonest example is, however, benign: the theca cell tumour. This tumour usually includes a prominent fibrous component, hence called a thecoma-fibroma, being dense, hard and rounded.

Germ Cell Tumours

These tumours show great variety (Table 6.6), being derived from totipotential cells. The commonest example is the benign teratoma. Its most prominent element is dermal, thus forming a cyst filled with sebum and hair (hence called a 'dermoid cyst'), but it commonly includes bone, cartilage and dental structures. Occasionally endocrine tissue, particularly thyroid, can cause hormonal disorder. Dermoid cysts commonly occur in young women. Although they occur rarely in young girls they account for the majority of ovarian tumours at that age.

All other germ cell tumours are malignant. Amongst this group, dysgerminomas are the most common; they need to be distinguished because they are very radiosensitive. Endodermal sinus tumours (of yolk-sac origin) and choriocarcinoma are very rare, but they need to be distinguished because they are highly sensitive to chemotherapy; they also secrete specific substances (alphafetoprotein and HCG, respectively) which can be used as tumour markers to monitor response to treatment.

Connective Tissue Tumours
These are uncommon. Indeed most 'fibromas' are probably thecoma-fibromas.

Metastatic Tumours
These comprise about 3 per cent of ovarian neoplasms, are often bilateral and usually originate from gastrointestinal carcinomas, being blood-borne.

Clinical Features of Benign Ovarian Tumours
Benign ovarian tumours occur at all ages, and of those occurring in young women about half are follicular cysts. They may remain 'silent' until they reach a very large size, when actual abdominal swelling and tightness of clothing is noticed. However, they are frequently brought to notice because of complications, which include:

physical accidents (commonest), all causing pain:
    torsion
    haemorrhage (into the tumour)
    rupture (of a cyst) leading to
        haemoperitoneum
        myxoma peritonei (in the case of mucinous cysts)
pressure symptoms
    pelvic discomfort
    urinary retention
endocrine/menstrual disturbance
obstruction of labour
infection (of the tumour: blood-borne)
malignant change (20 per cent).

Ovarian tumours, especially cysts, are frequently complicated by physical accidents, which all cause sudden pain. Torsion is the commonest and is most likely to affect medium-sized tumours, i.e. about 8–10 cm in diameter. The whole ovary and Fallopian tube twist about the broad ligament, strangulating the ovary and causing sudden severe pain and often vomiting. This may occur intermittently but, if it goes too far, congestion, oedema, haemorrhage and infarction of the ovary and tube occur, causing continuous severe pain and signs of peritonism. The main differential diagnosis is a bleeding ectopic pregnancy, but the ovarian mass is usually easily distinguished and in either case laparotomy is needed.

Rupture of a cyst causes bleeding and may also lead to widespread peritoneal seeding of neoplastic cells with malignant potential. In the case of mucinous cysts, even when benign, this can lead to a serious condition called myxoma peritonei – a form of mucinous ascites often associated with intestinal adhesions and obstruction.

Treatment

Ovarian tumours should always be excised without delay, for two main reasons: the high risk of malignancy or progression to malignancy, and the even higher risk of accident, particularly torsion, which is likely to disrupt or infarct the ovary and require its surgical sacrifice.

In premenopausal women, a discrete cystic swelling of the ovary up to 8 cm diameter is likely to be follicular, and its removal can be delayed for 6 weeks in the hope of regression.

In pregnancy, removal of a discrete cyst is better postponed until the middle trimester to minimize the risk of causing abortion.

In premenopausal women, cysts should be ennucleated, conserving the ovary. Rupture should be carefully avoided in case neoplastic cells are disseminated in the abdomen.

If there is any doubt whether an ovarian tumour is benign, the whole ovary should be removed and a frozen section of the tumour examined microscopically with a view to proceeding surgically for carcinoma (*see below*).

After the age of 40 bilateral oophorectomy with hysterectomy is best, because the tumour is always neoplastic, more likely to be malignant than in a young woman and reproductive function is not required.

Ovarian Cancer

Ovarian cancers are mainly of epithelial origin (i.e. carcinoma: serous, mucinous and endometrioid adenocarcinomas). Of the remainder the most likely types are dysgerminoma and granulosa cell and metastatic tumours.

Ovarian cancer occurs mostly after the menopause but is not uncommon between 30 and 40 years of age (*see Fig.* 6.1). It will occur in about 1 per cent of all women. It accounts for a quarter of all genital tract cancers but half the associated deaths (*see* Table 6.2). The relatively poor survival rate is due to the late clinical presentation of ovarian cancer; in about two-thirds of cases it has already spread beyond the pelvis.

Unfortunately there is no reliable means of screening for ovarian cancer. All that can be done towards early detection of neoplasms at their benign stage is to take every opportunity to do bimanual pelvic examination when vaginal examination is being performed, e.g. to take a cervical smear, at contraceptive clinics and at the antenatal 'booking' examination.

Spread occurs usually in the following order:

local invasion within pelvis
peritoneal seeding across the abdominal cavity
lymphatic embolization (*see Fig.* 2.8) to
    para-aortic nodes
    uterus
    other ovary
blood-borne metastasis.

The common presenting features are:

abdominal swelling due to a mass and/or ascites
abdominal pain
vaginal bleeding.

It is also not uncommon to find symptomless ovarian cancer accidentally.

Table 6.8. Clinical staging of ovarian cancer, required treatment and resulting success.

Stage	Treatment	5-year survival rate (corrected) %
1. Confined to ovary (i) unilateral, intact capsule	Cystectomy or unilateral oophorectomy and biopsy other ovary	60–90
(ii) bilateral, tumour excrescences	BSO, hysterectomy and omenectomy; with or without chemotherapy or intraperitoneal irradiation	
2. Extension within pelvis	As for stage 1, plus pelvic beam irradiation	40
3. Extension to abdominal peritoneum	Chemotherapy after surgery, as possible	10
4. Extension outside abdomen	As for stage 3, plus ?immunotherapy	1

BSO = bilateral salpingo-oophorectomy.

Treatment

This depends mainly on the extent of spread of the tumour, as shown in Table 6.8. There remains much controversy, however, about the choice of treatment, whether to be more or less aggressive. When the tumour capsule is intact (and the diagnosis of cancer may only be made later on histology) excellent results have been claimed for conservative surgery, which is particularly appropriate in young women, but this is not universally accepted. Chemotherapy is of course unpleasant and dangerous, and it is generally agreed that in advanced cancer it only achieves temporary remission, not eradication, of the disease; furthermore, surgical reduction of most of the tumour bulk is essential to give chemotherapy (or radiotherapy) a reasonable chance to be effective. It is therefore a difficult question in advanced ovarian cancer whether to seek the probably limited benefit from aggressive treatment or to take a fatalistic view and merely ease the patient's remaining passage through life.

Causes of death are commonly:

cachexia;
haemorrhage;
ureteric obstruction and renal failure;
intestinal obstruction.

Immunotherapy, using for example infusions of lymphocytes from pigs immunized with the particular cancer, is a future possibility now being explored.

As previously mentioned, dysgerminomas are best treated by radiotherapy, and the rare endodermal sinus tumour and choriocarcinoma by chemotherapy, following surgical 'bulk reduction' of the tumour.

Further Reading
Burghardt E. (1973) *Early Histological Diagnosis of Cervical Cancer*. Philadelphia, Saunders.
Coppleson M., Pixley E. and Reid B. (1978) *Colposcopy: a Scientific and Practical Approach to the Cervix and Vagina in Health and Disease*, 2nd ed. Springfield, Ill., Thomas.
Fox H. and Langley F. A. (1973) *Postgraduate Obstetrical and Gynaecological Pathology*. Oxford, Pergamon Press.
Kolstad P. and Stafl A. (1977) *Atlas of Colposcopy*, 2nd ed. Baltimore, University Park Press.
Langley F. A. (ed.) (1976) *Cancer of the Vulva, Vagina and Uterus. Clinics in Obstetrics and Gynaecology*, 3, (2). Eastbourne, Saunders.
Macnaughton M. C. and Govan A. D. T. (ed.) (1976) *The Ovary. Clinics in Obstetrics and Gynaecology*, 3, (1). Eastbourne, Saunders.
Waterhouse J. A. H. (1974) *Cancer Handbook of Epidemiology and Prognosis*. Edinburgh, Churchill Livingstone.

Chapter seven

Sexual Function

The physiological response to sexual stimulation follows the same pattern in the male and female, a four-stage response described by Masters and Johnson: (1) excitement, (2) plateau, (3) orgasm and (4) resolution. The length of each phase and the progression to the next depends on the efficacy of the stimulation on both the physical and emotional plane. The female is potentially multiorgasmic, that is she can return from the early resolution phase to the orgasmic repeatedly, provided stimulation is adequate. The male, however, is refractory to stimulation after orgasm and cannot return to orgasm until the refractory period has passed — a variable time which increases with age and varies with the individual from a few minutes to several hours.

Each phase is accompanied by general body and specific genital changes. Briefly the major changes are as follows (*Fig.* 7.1).

During the excitement phase there is general vasocongestion with erection of the penis and lubrication of the vagina. During the plateau phase there is engorgement of the lower third of the vagina and ballooning (or barrelling) of the upper two-thirds. During orgasm there are marked cardiorespiratory changes with the respiratory rate rising, pulse rates up to 180 per minute, and an increase in blood pressure of 20 mm Hg or more. At this time passive myotonic contractions of the buttocks and limbs occur, and the pelvic floor contracts involuntarily at 0·8-second intervals involving the anal sphincter, the vagina and urethra. A red mottling appears over the upper chest and neck which may be associated with a filmy sheen. This is the sex flush which varies with the intensity of the orgasm and fades very gradually during the resolution phase as the other changes subside.

Normal Sexual Intercourse

Normal sexual intercourse may be defined as anything erotic which gives pleasure to both partners, who are consenting adults, and does not hurt anyone. Any position which affords pleasure and satisfaction to both partners is to be considered normal, and experimentation is to be encouraged.

PLATEAU PHASE
Female   Male

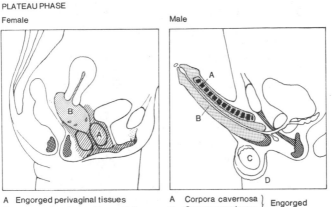

A Engorged perivaginal tissues   A Corpora cavernosa ⎱ Engorged
B Ballooned vagina and transudate   B Corpus spongiosum ⎰
                                       C Testes enlarge, engorge and rise
                                       D Dartos muscle thickened and contracted

Fig. 7.1. Plateau and orgasmic male and female organs.
(Redrawn from Helen Singer Kaplan's *The New Sex Therapy*, by kind
permission of Ballière Tindall, London, 1974.)

ORGASM

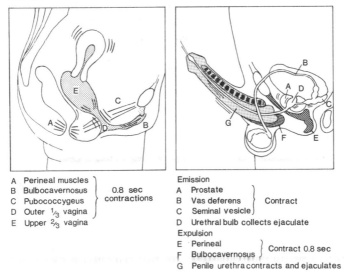

A Perineal muscles ⎫
B Bulbocavernosus ⎬ 0.8 sec
C Pubococcygeus   ⎭ contractions
D Outer ⅓ vagina
E Upper ⅔ vagina

Emission
A Prostate   ⎫
B Vas deferens   ⎬ Contract
C Seminal vesicle⎭
D Urethral bulb collects ejaculate
Expulsion
E Perineal   ⎫ Contract 0.8 sec
F Bulbocavernosus⎭
G Penile urethra contracts and ejaculates

If by normal sexual intercourse is meant the process of sexual intercourse as it is practised by the majority of adult humans then the following
is a description of the normal, but it has to be re-emphasized that there is
an enormous variation, and anything that is pleasurable to both partners

may be considered normal. The initiative is usually taken by the male, who indicates by looks, gestures, words and touching that he is sexually aroused. Foreplay involves touching, stroking, kissing and stimulating erotic areas, first in non-genital areas and later focusing on the genitals. The clitoris in the female is usually a vital receptor of stimulation, and accurate knowledge of its anatomy as well as communication about its function between partners may be the factor which decides the achievement of orgasm.

The aroused female may be aware of vaginal lubrication and may indeed reach orgasm without genital stimulation. Such reaction is quite normal in a minority who can climax from nipple stimulation or even fantasy. Towards the end of the excitement phase the female lies on her back, having removed at least her lower garments, and the male then lies above her (the missionary' position). Penile—vaginal contact is most readily made if the female takes the penis in one hand and separates her labia with the other, thus guiding the penis directly into the vagina. The male then thrusts up and down the vagina without withdrawing, the thrusting movements increasing in frequency as the orgasmic phase is approached. The female may have achieved orgasm before the male, or at the same time as the male. The male may continue thrusting during his orgasm and indeed afterwards, enabling the female who has not achieved orgasm to reach the orgasmic phase, or achieve a second or third orgasm. However, if unaware of the multiorgastic potential of his mate, the male may just maintain a deep vaginal entrenchment during his orgasm followed by detumescence during the resolution phase, perhaps leaving her unsatisfied.

There is no reason why manual stimulation of the clitoris should not be used at this stage to bring the female to orgasm. It is in the warmth of the shared resolution phase that the emotional relationship may be deepened. Without this special time the female may feel used or left out, thus beginning the emotional cycle which prevents eager anticipation of the next act of intercourse, and eventually leads to frigidity and impotence.

Since normal sex has been defined as anything which gives pleasure to both partners, for some this will mean a homosexual relationship, usually male, but as homosexuality is better understood and accepted, lesbianism presents more often and is also becoming more acceptable. For others this means oral and/or anal intercourse (although the latter is still illegal), both of which are in common use in a minority of partnerships. For some indulging in fetishes — that is acting out fantasies with leather, plastic and clothing, or in sadism and masochism, that is production of pain to one's partner and/or oneself — may play a major part in providing sexual stimulation. The increasing desire for these practices by one partner when the other finds them unacceptable presents the greatest of problems in attempting to decide where 'normality' lies and where adjustments can be made. The doctor must always keep in mind the vast range of normality and the many factors influencing sexual function when faced with sexual problems.

Masturbation

The response follows the same pattern regardless of the source of stimulation. The orgasm achieved by masturbation is identical in physiological terms to that achieved by hetero- or homosexual coitus, although the emotional content may alter the way orgasm is perceived. Masturbation is a normal sexual function releasing sexual tensions and in a modified degree it is an almost universal infancy and childhood experience. Only a minority of persons do not masturbate by the time they reach the age of 20. Women are slower to discover masturbation and it is not until their forties that numbers begin to equilibrate, but the Kinsey Report and others have shown that at all ages more men than women masturbate. Masturbation is completely harmless and unrelated to blindness, venereal disease, sterility and any infirmity. There is no evidence to suggest that it causes labial hypertrophy any more than that it makes the penis drop off.

Sexual Function in a Loving Relationship

Coitus is only part of a loving relationship (*Fig.* 7.2) but may disrupt that relationship if dysfunction occurs. If a husband is disliked, or equally if a wife poses a threat to her partner, orgasmic dysfunction may result.

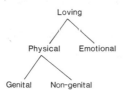

Fig. 7.2. Sexual function in a loving relationship.

Factors Affecting Sexual Function

1. *Childhood experience:* This affects adult sexuality and is linked with unconscious motivation and the Oedipus-Electra conflict.

2. *Partner rejection:* An unsuitable relationship with partner rejection and failure to communicate is clearly unlikely to be associated with good sexual function.

3. *Ignorance and inadequate techniques:* Satisfactory sexual function depends on both partners receiving adequate stimulation and being free to respond to this. Ignorance may lead to sexual anxiety and fears of failure. In the male this may cause premature ejaculation which enhances the fear of failure and may lead to impotence; in the female such fears, often allied to inadequate understanding of the clitoral stimulation and communication about this in a partnership, cause a dry vagina, dyspareunia and eventually frigidity.

4. *Disease:* General ill health and chronic pain decrease libido in both sexes. Long-standing uncontrolled diabetes mellitus may be associated with partial impotence; vaginal or pelvic pathology may cause dyspareunia, and the pain experienced during intercourse leads to fear and rejection of coitus. Many other disorders alter sexual function, from the rigid limbs of the spastic to the problems following ileostomy. Chronic and progressive disease such as multiple sclerosis poses a special problem because genital sensation disappears in the female. A couple may be helped to understand the pleasure of oral sex and so prolong a happy sexual relationship.

5. *Pregnancy:* Many women find intercourse more enjoyable during pregnancy and achieve orgasm more readily at this time. Patients should have intercourse during pregnancy whenever they wish. It is, however, usual practice to ask the patient who has a history of recurrent abortion to refrain from intercourse around the time that she usually miscarries and also to advise abstinence in patients who have bled during the pregnancy. There is some suggestion that the uterine contractions provoked as a result of orgasm could be related to the onset of premature labour, and a patient with a history of premature labour may be advised to refrain from intercourse around her danger time.

6. *Drugs:* Drugs usually diminish rather than enhance sexual pleasure, and most aphrodisiacs are pharmacologically inactive. If they do enhance erotic behaviour it is by placebo effects. Small doses of alcohol, barbiturates and amphetamines may release inhibitions and apparently enhance sexuality, but chronic abuse of all of them causes sexual depression. Impotence is a frequent complication of methylodopa, and many other drugs also depress sexual function.

Sexual Dysfunction

Male

Male sexual dysfunction falls into three main groups: (1) impotence, (2) premature ejaculation and (3) retardation or failure of ejaculation. Impotence and premature ejaculation are such very common problems that they may be regarded as part of normal male sexuality, provided that they do not persist.

Impotence: Rarely, this may be of pathological or physiological origin. The prerequisites of erection are intact erectile tissue with an adequate blood supply and intact innervation to the penis. Pathological impotence results from faults at these points. Psychological factors are the cause of failure of erection, or loss of erection at any time during the excitement or plateau phase. Such problems often apply to a man only in a specific partnership; he may find himself entirely normal in a casual rather than committed (or long-term) relationship.

Premature ejaculation: This is an extremely common problem which resolves spontaneously in most cases but not infrequently requires special therapy. The attitude of the partner is all important in order to prevent persistent premature ejaculation from developing into impotence.

Retardation or failure of ejaculation: Fears regarding performance and fears regarding pregnancy may prevent ejaculation. In later middle age pleasurable satisfactory intercourse without ejaculation is not uncommon. The number of times intercourse ends with ejaculation becomes less.

Female
Female sexual dysfunction is less obvious, but probably even more common. Fear of frigidity enhances and may even produce dysfunction.

General sexual dysfunction: The woman may be averse to sexual approaches. She will then fail to lubricate and show no genital engorgement. There is little or no vasocongestion in response to sexual stimulation.

Orgasmic dysfunction: Here lubrication occurs and there is evidence of vasocongestion, but there is failure to enjoy the responses to sexual stimulation and/or failure to reach orgasm. In some cases this may be regarded as a type of defence mechanism, the woman being afraid to 'let go'. It is important to differentiate between general sexual dysfunction and orgasmic dysfunction, as different therapies are required for treatment.

Treatment and Referral
The general practitioner must listen to what is said and not said, he must give the impression of having unlimited time and he must never show disapproval or censure. He must always exclude pathology, before assuming that causative factors are psychological.

Unless the family doctor has special training and wishes to undertake counselling and therapy himself, referral may be necessary.

Family Planning Clinics
Usually one or more doctors in any such clinic have had special training and hold special sessions during which psychosexual counselling is undertaken. Such special training is available to all doctors through the Institute of Psychosexual Medicine.

Marriage Guidance Council
This also offers the help of trained counsellors – usually not medically qualified but with some special training and virtually unlimited time.

Out-Patient Clinics
A general gynaecological or psychiatric clinic is NOT a place to which these patients should be referred unless there is specific gynaecologic or psychiatric pathology. Psychosexual counselling sessions may be carried out by gynaecologists or psychiatrists specially interested and trained in psychosexual therapy.

Sexual activity is just one of many normal body functions. You are trained to take a history about body functions so do not omit a history of sexual function. Give patients the opportunity to discuss their sexual function and problems; listen sympathetically and know where help may be obtained in your community.

Further Reading

Kaplan Helen Singer (1974) *The New Sex Therapy. Active Treatment of Sexual Dysfunctions.* London, Ballière Tindall.
Masters W. H. and Johnson V. E. (1966) *Human Sexual Response.* Boston, Little Brown.

Chapter eight

Contraception, Sterilization and Therapeutic Abortion

The demand for medical provision of contraception, sterilization and therapeutic abortion has increased dramatically in recent years, and each of these related topics will form a substantial part of the workload of most gynaecologists and general practitioners. Although sterilization operations will generally be performed in specialist units, they really form part of the range of contraceptive methods, and all doctors should be able to provide information to patients about sterilization as well as contraception. For the foreseeable future, contraceptive methods as well as patients are likely to remain fallible, and there will be a place for abortion as the long stop of family planning methods.

CONTRACEPTION

Four groups of contraceptive methods will be considered: (1) hormonal, (2) intrauterine devices, (3) barrier methods and (4) other methods. In the past (3) and (4) were the predominant methods, but recent years have seen a swing to the more reliable methods of the first two groups.

Hormonal Contraception

Oestrogen—Progestogen Combinations
With the exception of Minilyn (which has 22) all preparations contain 21 identical active pills containing oestrogen and progestogen. A few preparations have 7 additional inert pills.

Actions
The principal action is suppression of ovulation by interference with the pituitary ovarian system. Three secondary actions assist contraception:

1. Prevention of physiological cycle in the endometrium. It is not prepared for nidation of a blastocyst.
2. Inhibition of cervical mucus changes that normally encourage sperm migration.
3. Interference with ovum transport in the Fallopian tubes and uterus.

109

Formulation

Since the Scowen Committee Report in 1969 linking thromboembolic side-effects with higher doses of oestrogens, for practical purposes all combinations used include 50 micrograms or less of either ethinyloestradiol or mestranol. Mestranol has a lesser oestrogenic effect than ethinyloestradiol (approximately 60 per cent).

The progestogens are synthetic compounds varying widely in molecular structure and potency. Their action is similar to progesterone in that they induce progestational changes in the oestrogenized endometrium, but if used continuously they tend to inhibit endometrial growth altogether. The most commonly used progestogen is now norgestrel.

Method of Use

The pills are taken one daily for 21 (or 22) days with a gap between each pack of 7 (or 6) days. Protection against conception is continuous after the first 14 pills of the first pack if they are started on day 5 of the cycle, or immediately if started on day 1. Combined oral contraceptives may be started immediately after a termination or miscarriage, or 3 weeks after delivery. Protection continues if one pill is forgotten, provided it is taken within 24 hours in addition to the next day's pill. During the interval between packs there is usually, but not always, some uterine bleeding.

Hazards

Oestrogen–progestogen combinations can only be obtained on medical prescription as there are various hazards associated with their use. Some are mild, some very serious, but their prevalence is fortunately slight and certainly far less than most non-medical people believe. They are certainly small compared with the risk of an unwanted pregnancy. The major hazards are as follows.

THROMBOEMBOLISM

There is an increased incidence of leg vein thrombosis, pulmonary embolus and cerebral thrombosis produced by the oestrogen component of the pill. With the lower dose pills the mortality risk from these conditions is of the order of 1 per 100 000 women per year, less than a tenth of the risk associated with a pregnancy and small compared with the risk of smoking even a few cigarettes per day.

METABOLIC EFFECTS

Changes in virtually every aspect of metabolism have been recorded in pill users. These changes tend to alter the normal female metabolic pattern towards either the male pattern or that found in early pregnancy. Probably the most important of these changes is an increase in levels of cholesterol and other lipids, which almost certainly accounts for the observed slightly increased incidence of ischaemic heart disease in the older (over 30 years) long-term oral contraceptive user. Glucose tolerance is also reduced (as in pregnancy), very occasionally producing overt diabetes in a latent diabetic. All of these metabolic effects appear to be dose-related, and are minimal with the newer norgestrel-containing pills.

HYPERTENSION
The occasional patient gets a significant elevation of blood pressure while taking oral contraceptives.

DEPRESSION
A few patients will get quite severe depression while taking the pill. This has been shown to be related to disturbances in tryptophan metabolism, and is partly treatable by pyridoxine (Vitamin B_6).

Medical Care
Before prescribing oestrogen progestogen pills, the doctor should ensure as far as possible that there is no predisposition to thromboembolism which the pill might potentiate. Also, the medical history should identify disturbances of liver function, which might interfere with steroid metabolism, and the pre-existence of conditions such as migraine, the later occurrence of which might be ascribed to the pill.

An assessment must be made of any intercurrent illness or condition which might be affected by taking the pill. If necessary, specialist advice should be sought. Examples are: diabetes mellitus, essential hypertension, renal disease and psychiatric illnesses. It is important in making this assessment not to forget the possible harm resulting from further pregnancy.

The physical examination should include measurement of the body weight and blood pressure, and also exclude a carcinoma of the breast or cervix that might be adversely affected by administered sex steroids.

Women over 30 years should be discouraged from long-term pill usage if an acceptable alternative exists.

Choice of Preparation
The higher dose preparations give better cycle control and virtually always control dysmenorrhoea, but the associated metabolic disturbances and hazards are greater. The norgestrel-containing pills should probably be the initial choice.

Progestogen-only Pills
Actions
These are similar to those of oestrogen—progestogen combined pills except that ovulation is not reliably suppressed. They rely on:

1. Changes in the maturation of endometrium which inhibit implantation.

2. Constant hostility of cervical mucus to sperm that lasts throughout the cycle.
3. Interference with the tubal transport of ova.

Formulation
The dose of progestogen is lower than that in the combined pills, about one-third to one-tenth, and oestrogen is entirely absent.

Method of Use
The pills are supplied in packs of 28 or 42 and one is taken every day at roughly the same time of day. Note that there is no interval: the tablets are taken continuously.

Hazards and Medical Care
Adverse effects are very uncommon except for irregular uterine bleeding. This may be severe enough to prevent patients continuing. It usually settles to a more or less regular cycle after 6–9 months. Other problems are rare but include skin reactions, breast discomfort and occasional symptoms of 'premenstrual tension'.

ACCIDENTAL PREGNANCY
This is the most serious drawback to the use of progestogen-only pills. Rates reported vary considerably from 2 to 6 per 100 women years, and a disproportionate number of these pregnancies are ectopic.

INDICATIONS
Progestogen-only pills are suitable for patients who suffer adverse effects from pills containing oestrogen. They are also useful in lactation as milk supply is not affected.

DEPOT CONTRACEPTION
Progestogens have been used in depot form, given as an intramuscular injection (usually medroxyprogesterone acetate 150 mg or 300 mg in oil) to last 3–6 months. Irregular bleeding, or amenorrhoea with anovulation are common side-effects.

Postcoital Contraception
The aim is to inhibit implantation of the fertilized ovum by giving an oral dose of hormone. This form of contraception is not really suitable for long-term use, but can be useful as a 'first aid measure'.
    Either an abnormally high dose of an oestrogenic combined pill (e.g. Eugynon 50 tabs ii stat. and repeated after 12 hours) or progestogens (e.g. Femulen 0·5 mg tabs ii daily for 10 days) are effective.

Methods of Use
Patients should begin the treatment within 24 hours of unprotected intercourse.

Hazards and Medical Care
History taking should aim to exclude those in whom high oestrogens would be particularly hazardous (e.g. any predisposition to thrombo-embolism, any liver dysfunction). The exposure is brief and the risk of thromboembolism is not yet known. The effect on the fetus, if pregnancy occurs, is not known. In many cases termination of pregnancy would be advisable.

Intrauterine Devices (IUDs)

Inactive Devices
These are small objects made of polyethylene or nylon (previously gold or silver).

They are designed to fit into the uterine cavity and have various configurations. Usually the shape has led to the commonly-used name, e.g. 'shield', 'ring', 'coil', 'loop' (which is not a loop but a zig-zag shape), together often with the name of the inventor.

Many of the IUDs have one or two nylon threads fixed to the lower end which normally protrude from the cervical canal. These assist simple removal and also demonstrate the presence of the IUD in the uterine cavity.

Mode of Action
IUDs are considered to inhibit the implantation of the blastocyst in the endometrium, possibly by altering the pH of the uterine secretion thus inhibiting the essential enzymes. There is a small round-cell infiltration in the endometrium when an IUD is present but normally this does not proceed to full-scale inflammation. The mildness of the reaction is possibly due to the short length of time that the endometrium is in contact with the IUD before being shed in menstruation. Changes in tubal motility, possibly affecting egg transport, have also been demonstrated.

Effectiveness
The devices vary in their effectiveness against conception (from 1·5 per 100 women years for the Lippes Loop D, to 5·5 per 100 women years for the small Birnberg Bow). The important facts are that they are not as effective against pregnancy as combined oestrogen–progestogen pills, but there is much less chance of 'user-failure', e.g. by forgetting to take pills regularly or running out of supplies.

Complications and Side-Effects
IUDs may be a nearly perfect method of contraception for many patients,

but over a period of 2 years of use, about 30 per cent of Lippes Loops will have to be abandoned for reasons other than planned pregnancy. Removals are most common on account of:

1. *Bleeding.* Periods may be unduly heavy or prolonged. Less commonly there is constant intermenstrual bleeding. Iron deficiency anaemia can occur in women with IUDs, even without subjectively excessive losses.
2. *Pain.* In some patients uterine pains occur after insertion and gradually subside. In a small number the pains continue and are not tolerable.
3. *Expulsion.* If unnoticed, expulsion may lead to unplanned pregnancy.
4. *Pregnancy* with the device in the uterus ('accidental pregnancy').
5. *'At patient's request'.* A small number of patients ask for their IUD to be removed after a time, for no apparently logical reason. Others may simply wish to change their contraceptive method.
6. *Infection.* Occasionally tubal or intrauterine infection occurs. Most cases can be treated with the device in. If there is not a good response immediately or the infection is initially severe, the IUD should be removed.

Insertion

In most parous women, insertion of an intrauterine device is an easy outpatient procedure. If there is any substantial difficulty the operator should not continue the attempt. It can always be carried out at another time under theatre conditions, if necessary with a general anaesthetic, or a local intracervical block.

In nulliparous women, insertion is more difficult and painful and the side-effects in use more severe.

After insertion, hypotension and bradycardia may occur, even if insertion has been very easy. All patients should not leave for 10 minutes and be able to lie down if necessary.

IUDs should never be inserted in the presence of pelvic inflammatory disease.

Perforation of the uterus is a rare complication following insertion.

At present there is no evidence to suggest that inactive IUDs need to be replaced routinely unless they cause symptoms.

Active Intrauterine Devices
Background

Owing to poor long-term continuity rates with inactive devices, attempts have been made to incorporate active antifertility agents in smaller IUDs.

Active agents used so far are metals and hormones. Virgin copper wire has been used very successfully in the Endouterine T (Copper-T) and Graviguard (Copper-7) and Multiload devices.

Progesterone was tried in a T-device (Progestasert). This had the advantage of a low pregnancy rate and a lower incidence of bleeding problems, but it was relatively large and difficult to insert, needed to be changed annually, was very expensive and had a high ectopic pregnancy rate.

Insertion
Insertion of the small devices is much easier for the patient. The Copper-7 introducer is only 3 mm in external diameter. This allows it to be a feasible method for women who have never been pregnant, in contrast to the inactive devices. Results of its use in nulliparous women are good. Care is required in inserting the Copper-7, to ensure that the transverse limb reaches the fundus of the uterus in a full open position.

Perforation is rare, but there is a marked omental reaction to a Copper-7 device in the peritoneal cavity, and misplaced devices should be removed within a few days. This is usually possible through a laparoscope.

Mode of Action
The small plastic shape alone has very little contraceptive effect. The action of copper and similar metals is not certainly known, but traces of copper ions are known to inhibit enzymes, such as alkaline phosphatase which may be required for implantation. Cupric ions are toxic to sperm in lower mammals.

Effectiveness
The copper devices are highly effective against pregnancy, giving accidental pregnancy rates of between 1 and 2 per 100 women years.

Complications and Side-Effects
These are of the same kind as those of other IUDs, but removals for bleeding and pains are greatly reduced with the copper devices because of their smaller size.

The copper is not significantly absorbed systemically, and in the case of accidental pregnancy the evidence suggests that there is no danger from teratogenicity. All active agents are slowly lost by elution, and active devices require replacement at intervals. Replacement of the copper devices is recommended every 2 or 3 years.

Pregnancy with an IUD
A relatively high proportion of pregnancies occurring with an IUD in situ will be ectopic pregnancies (although the absolute rate of ectopic pregnancy probably does not exceed that in the general population). Dalkon Shields (in situ) have been shown to be associated with a high rate of middle trimester septic abortion, and should be removed routinely if present in early pregnancy. All coils (in situ in pregnancy) are associated

with a high spontaneous abortion rate, and probably a higher late pregnancy complication rate.

Barrier Methods

Mode of Action
Barrier appliances are designed to prevent the direct insemination of the cervical mucus with spermatozoa. They are used with spermicidal substances which are placed so as to be in direct contact with the seminal fluid in the vagina.

The Condom, Sheath or 'French Letter'
This is rolled on to the erect penis before coitus and retains the ejaculated semen. Spermicides are not always used with condoms, but if so they increase their effectiveness, reduce the risk of them bursting and help to lubricate them.

The Diaphragm or 'Dutch Cap'
This is the most commonly used and probably the safest (against pregnancy) female barrier method. It fits like a ring pessary between the posterior fornix and the anterior vaginal wall just above the symphysis pubis. It is not as heavily constructed as a ring pessary and is surprisingly unobtrusive during coitus if correctly fitted. The woman places it in the vagina herself before coitus and it must remain in position for at least 8 hours afterwards. The correct size is estimated by a doctor or specially trained nurse, and the patient is carefully instructed in the correct manner of use. In fitting a diaphragm it is important to ensure (1) that the cervix is covered, (2) that the lower edge fits snugly into the sulcus above the symphysis and (3) that the width of the vagina is filled at the cervical level without causing undue lateral stretch, leading to ridging of the posterior vaginal wall. Most women take a 70–75 mm cap. Routine checks of fit should be made, initially after a week and then every 6 months. Variation is caused by age, pregnancy, change in pelvic muscle tone and change in intrapelvic fat tissue related to changes in body weight.

The Cervical Cap
This fits tightly over the cervix but otherwise is used in the same way as the diaphragm. Its use requires that the cervix is of a suitable shape, and it is slightly more difficult to manipulate than the diaphragm.

The Vault Cap
This is an intravaginal cap, made of firmer rubber than the diaphragm and the cervical cap, which fits across the cervix and adheres by suction to the fornices. It is designed for use by women who have insufficient tone in the pelvic floor to hold a diaphragm in place but whose cervix is not suitable for a cervical cap.

The 'Vimule' Cap
This is a vault cap with a central projection to contain a long cervix.

Effectiveness
It has been said that the use of a barrier and spermicide by a well-motivated couple gives results at least as good against pregnancy as an intrauterine device, and without the problematical side-effects. The crucial factor is motivation, with perseverance in correct use, and it is often in this that the method breaks down. Many people find caps and condoms 'messy' and inconvenient by comparison with their expectations from more up-to-date methods, and will fail to use them on every occasion. This means that the general figures obtained from studying their use often give high rates of failure. Overall pregnancy rates of around 5 per cent per year can be expected.

Other Methods
All other methods are relatively inefficient, with pregnancy rates probably in excess of 10 per 100 women years in general use.

Coitus Interruptus (Withdrawal)
Here the male aims to withdraw his penis from the vagina just before ejaculation occurs. The method fails not infrequently because he may not possess the necessary degree of control, because some sperm may leak before the main ejaculation occurs, and because semen deposited on the vulva may still allow a pregnancy to occur.

The Safe Period (Rhythm Method)
Pregnancy is only likely to occur in the few days leading up to ovulation. The safe period method relies on estimating when this is likely to be, and avoiding coitus during that time. The reliability of the method can be increased by recording the basal temperature, to give a closer estimate of ovulation timing. However, it has been reliably shown that sperms can survive for 8 days in preovulatory mucus and precise prediction of the ovulation date is, in practice, difficult.

Chemicals
A number of pessaries, creams, foams and other chemical preparations have been produced for use as sole contraceptive agents. The results are so poor that they cannot be recommended, except as adjuncts to the barrier methods.

STERILIZATION
The use of male and female sterilization for social rather than medical indications has only been widespread since the late 1960s, but it now forms a major part of the world's contraceptive efforts. It is estimated that

in the USA 1 million sterilization operations are carried out annually, and 20 per cent of all married couples have had one partner sterilized.

Female Sterilization

This may be performed laparoscopically, though a small suprapubic incision, or through an incision in the posterior vaginal fornix. Laparoscopically the tubes may be occluded by diathermy or by applying clips or plastic rings. Diathermy carries some risk of bowel damage. The umbilical incision leave no significant scar, and hospital stay is brief, some surgeons using local anaesthesia and discharging the patient the same day.

At open operation a wide variety of techniques for tubal ligation may be employed. With the Pomeroy method a knuckle of tube is tied and excised on each side, while the Oxford technique separates the cut ends of the tubes by the round ligament in order to minimize the possibility of recanalization. Hospital stay is longer but serious side-effects are less common than with the laparoscopic approach. Through the posterior fornix the tubes are diathermized or a simple ligation technique used. The complication rate and hospital stay is comparable to that of laparoscopic sterilization.

Failure Rate

About 3 or 4 per 1000 women can be expected to become pregnant after a Pomeroy tubal ligation. Failure rates for laparoscopic or culdoscopic (posterior fornix) sterilization are similar, depending on the experience of the operator. The more sophisticated tubal ligation methods such as the Oxford technique have failure rates of 1 per 1000 or less.

Reversibility

Female sterilization may be reversed with 50 per cent or better success, as long as minimal amounts of tube were destroyed by the original operation. Simple ligation without removal of a segment of tube, or laparoscopic clip sterilization are the most reversible techniques.

Side-Effects

Apart from operation complications, side-effects are rare. There is no real evidence for the common belief that female sterilization causes menstrual problems.

Male Sterilization – Vasectomy

This is a simple procedure that can be done under local anaesthesia. The vas is divided and tied off through small scrotal incisions. Sperm are still produced in the ejaculate for several months afterwards, and continued contraception with semen examination starting at 3 and 4 months after operation and continuing until the ejaculate is sperm-free is essential.

Failure Rate
As long as adequate follow-up procedures are employed, failures should be less than 1 per 1000.

Complications
Haematoma formation and local infection may occur in occasional cases.

Reversibility
Vasectomy can be successfully reversed in approximately 50 per cent of cases. Removal of more than 2 cm vas, or removal of the convoluted part of the vas limit success.

Counselling for Sterilization
Both partners should be seen together. The choice of which partner to sterilize will usually be determined by the attitudes of the couple, and it is rarely profitable to persuade them otherwise. A simple explanation of the procedure and any follow-up routine should be given. Some enquiry into their sexual stability should be made. Sterilization should have no effect on a normal sex life, but is no cure for sexual problems and may in fact aggravate them. The procedure should be presented as basically irreversible, and the possible circumstances that could lead them to regret their decision should be fully discussed.

ABORTION
The 1967 Abortion Act made abortion legal in the UK in the following circumstances:

1. The continuance of the pregnancy would involve risk to the life of the pregnant woman greater than if the pregnancy were terminated.
2. The continuance of the pregnancy would involve risk of injury to the physical or mental health of the pregnant woman greater than if the pregnancy were terminated.
3. The continuance of the pregnancy would involve risk of injury to the physical or mental health of the existing child(ren) of the family of the pregnant woman greater than if the pregnancy were terminated.
4. There is a substantial risk that if the child were born it would suffer from such physical or mental abnormalities as to be seriously handicapped.

Two doctors are required to certify that one of these clauses applies to the woman concerned. Over 100 000 legal abortions are performed in this country annually.

Aspiration Termination
The cervix is dilated in proportion to the size of the uterus. The uterus is then evacuated with a suction curette. This technique is relatively safe and simple until 12 weeks. Up to 8 weeks aspiration termination can

be done with a local anaesthetic, and this is the safest of all methods of termination.

Late Termination

After 12 weeks aspiration termination is hazardous. Abortion may be induced with prostaglandins either extra-amniotically (introduced through a cervical catheter) or intra-amniotically (introduced by amniocentesis). Intra-amniotic hypertonic saline, and hysterotomy are more hazardous and now rarely used.

Hysterectomy

There may be a place for hysterectomy in the older parous woman with menstrual problems or pelvic pathology.

Complications

Serious complications are rare and termination before 12 weeks carries less risk than a term pregnancy, but the following may occur:

Incomplete abortion with subsequent sepsis or haemorrhage.
Sensitization of Rh-negative women (give anti-D — *see* Chapter 13).
Cervical damage leading to subsequent middle trimester abortion (mainly if cervix dilated more than 10 Hegar).
Uterine perforation.

Further Reading

Handbook of the International Planned Parenthood Federation (1979) Vol. 13, No. 5 London, IPPF.
Hawkins D. F. and Elder M. G. (1979) *Human Fertility Control: Theory and Practice.* London, Butterworth.
Peel J. and Potts D. M. (1969) *Textbook of Contraceptive Practice.* (Illustrated.) Cambridge, Cambridge University Press.

Chapter nine

Gynaecological Disorders of Childhood, Puberty and the Menopause

CHILDHOOD

Genital problems are uncommon and mostly trivial, but one of the rarest — abnormal sexual differentiation — is profoundly important and easily overlooked. Tumours are extremely rare (*see* Chapter 6).

In the newborn girl vaginal bleeding or breast engorgement and secretion ('witch's milk') may occur due to the previous stimulation by placental hormones, but it is transient.

Vaginal bleeding in young girls may be due to sarcoma botryoides of the cervix, to urethral prolapse or trauma. Trauma is often self-inflicted by a sharp object out of curiosity. Since the vaginal vault might have been penetrated it is important to examine the abdomen in case of peritoneal bleeding or peritonitis.

Vaginal discharge in young girls is usually bacterial, unlike in the young adult, and sometimes due to the presence of a small foreign body — often long forgotten — in the vagina. Speculum examination may, therefore, be necessary and can only be successfully done under general anaesthesia. Often the cause is bad hygiene — not only due to neglect but also misplaced fastidiousness — which is easily corrected.

Abnormal Sexual Differentiation ('Intersex')

In practice this is defined as indeterminate external (phenotypic) gender. Gender can be defined in chromosomal, gonadal, phenotypic or psychological terms, but in children it is abnormality of the external genitalia that presents itself. The abnormality may not be recognized and so the gender may be interpreted wrongly with respect to the chromosomal and gonadal gender, i.e. pseudohermaphroditism. The mistake will only become apparent at puberty with disastrous consequences for the individual because of the need for plastic operations and, worse, the psychological upheaval necessary to change her accustomed gender. If these tragedies are to be avoided it is extremely important to examine the external genitalia at birth with great care, and deal with any abnormality early.

Every degree of abnormality is possible, but for illustration only the most typical, i.e. extreme, examples will be described.

121

Female pseudohermaphroditism   means female chromosomal and gonadal gender associated with apparently male external genitalia. It can be caused by administration of androgens, including some progestogens, to the mother pregnant with a female fetus. More commonly it is due to congenital adrenal hyperplasia in which there is excessive androgen production by the female fetus's adrenal cortex due to any of a variety of enzymic defects which block the synthetic pathway for cortisol. The precursors and androgen side-products are secreted in excess because the cortisol deficiency leads to excessive secretion of ACTH. The fetus may be partly protected, however, by maternal cortisol which crosses the placenta, and masculinization may only occur later. At birth there is likely to be clitoral enlargement and a cloacal membrane, resembling a boy with hypospadias and undescended testicles (*see Fig.* 2.3*b,c*). In some cases the baby's life is endangered by a salt-losing syndrome due to associated aldosterone deficiency.

Male pseudohermaphroditism   means male chromosomal and gonadal gender but with apparently female external genitalia. The testicles are undescended, often intra-abdominal, and the vulva may be typically female, but the vagina is absent or short, and the uterus is missing. The abnormality may be recognized at birth only by separating the labia and looking for the (absent) shadowy depth of the normal vaginal canal. Congenital inguinal hernias are often also present. If overlooked the problem will present at puberty with clitoral enlargement and deepening voice due to testosterone. However, a similar abnormality, testicular feminization, may be due to insensitivity to androgens (on the part of all normally responsive tissues), whether the androgens are of testicular or adrenal origin, so masculinization does not occur nor does axillary and pubic hair grow (*see* Puberty, *below*). The testicles secrete normal amounts of hormones. In the fetus, Müllerian inhibiting substance prevents development of the uterus and upper vagina. At puberty there is enough oestradiol to induce otherwise normal secondary female differentiation (of breasts and body fat). Thus the individual presents usually as an apparent girl with delayed menarche.

True hermaphroditism,   in which there is a testicle and ovary, or ovotestes, with mixed development of the internal and external genitalia, is extremely rare.

Management of intersex depends on the age at which it is recognized. Once the child is accustomed to its gender it is usually better not changed, but a female pseudohermaphrodite with very inadequate external male differentiation may well be better converted from the accustomed male gender. Psychological factors are most important. Whatever the age at discovery, it is essential to define the exact genital configuration by examination under anaesthesia and laparoscopy and/or laparotomy.

Abdominal testicles should be excised because of the risk of developing dysgerminoma in later life, and oestrogen therapy will be required at the age of puberty. Cosmetic surgery on the external genitalia may be necessary, and later the young adult 'woman' will usually require a functional vagina constructed.

PUBERTY AND ADOLESCENCE
Puberty

The proper meaning of puberty is procreative capability but the word is usually applied to the events leading up to this state. Thus in this book puberty is taken to be the time of development of the genitalia and secondary sexual characters leading up to the menarche (first menstruation). The time of further maturation to adulthood is adolescence.

The Events of Puberty

1. The neuroendocrinological changes that initiate all the other recognizable events of puberty are imperfectly understood, but are clearly the result of maturation of the hypothalamus rather than of any primary change in the gonads. The changes involve the adrenocortical as well as the gonadal axis, and occur gradually from early childhood. The maturation of the hypothalamus in terms of gonadotrophin releasing hormone secretion seems to depend on pheromones. Gonadotrophin secretion by the anterior pituitary increases steadily from early childhood, and the sensitivity of ovarian response is enhanced by oestrogens produced by subcutaneous fat from adrenocortical precursors. Thus body weight, especially fat weight, partly determines the age of puberty, and menarche occurs on average at 47 kg (7½ stones) – although the range is wide. Increased secretion of adrenocortical androgens is responsible for many of the events of puberty – the body growth spurt and axillary and pubic hair growth – which are thus called 'adrenarche'. The further differential growth of bone, muscle and fat, effecting the typical body shapes of men and women is due to the additional secretion by the gonads of testosterone or oestradiol respectively.
2. Breast development (thelarche) is the first externally noticeable change, starting at 11 years on average (normal range 9–13 years), and takes longest (up to 5 years) to complete.
3. Pubic hair growth usually starts next, together with:
4. Growth of genital organs.
5. Body growth accelerates, reaching peak velocity about 11 months before menarche, with remarkable constancy in the relative timing of these two events.
6. Menarche occurs at 13 years on average (normal range 11–15 years).
7. Axillary hair growth may start before or after menarche.

Adolescence

This is the time from menarche to adulthood when physical, mental and reproductive maturation occurs. The physical and reproductive events that occur are:

1. Further slow growth in body height for 3—4 years until closure of epiphyses due to androgens and oestrogens.
2. Further maturation of breasts and labia.
3. Main growth of axillary hair.
4. Regularization of menstrual cycle and gradually increased frequency of ovulation up to about 20 years. This is not to say that the fertility of adolescent girls is low!

Problems of Puberty and Adolescence

The most common problems are due to inadequate sex education, but the deficiency applies less to the physical aspects, more often to the development of interpersonal relationships, love and the value of sex. For these reasons venereal disease, contraceptive problems, pregnancy and the need for abortion are becoming rapidly more common at this age.

Reproductive disorders particularly associated with puberty and adolescence include:

1. Primary or secondary amenorrhoea or oligomenorrhoea (*see* following section and Chapter 10).
2. Dysfunctional (excessive) uterine bleeding (*see* Chapter 5).
3. Spasmodic dysmenorrhoea (*see* Chapter 3).
4. Abnormal sex differentiation (*see above*).
5. Precocious puberty, very rarely (*see below*).

Delayed Puberty and Menarche

Delayed puberty means failure of development of all the secondary sexual characteristics including menarche. Although it could be recognized as early as 14 years by failure of breast development, it is not usually accepted as such till menstruation has been delayed too (i.e. at 16 years). The cause is nearly always primary failure of one of the components of the hypothalamic-pituitary-ovarian axis:

1. Primary hypothalamic failure may be temporary (true delayed puberty, which will resolve spontaneously) or permanent (Kallman's syndrome, which is associated with hyposmia, i.e. impaired sense of smell, and presumably impaired reception of pheromones).
2. Primary pituitary failure is rare, and then usually due to a large pituitary tumour or a craniopharyngioma compressing the pituitary or its stalk.
3. Primary ovarian failure due to ovarian dysgenesis is the commonest cause of delayed puberty. The ovaries are typically mere 'streaks' of

tissue without any follicles, and although classically associated with Turner's syndrome, often no abnormality can be found except for the ovaries. In the latter cases it is assumed that there is a mosaic chromosomal abnormality affecting only the ovaries.

Anorexia nervosa and hyperprolactinaemia causing secondary failure of the ovarian axis (see Chapter 10) rarely occur early enough to interfere with puberty.

In all these cases, apart from any specific treatment that might be appropriate, the need for oestrogen replacement therapy must be carefully considered because premature epiphyseal closure can occur as a result.

Delayed menarche means failure to menstruate by 16 years. It may or may not be associated with other delayed pubertal development (*see above*). When secondary sexual development otherwise appears normal the causes may be:

1. Atresia of the vagina or cervix, resulting in retention of the normal menses (cryptomenorrhoea). Most commonly the atresia is lower vaginal and very limited. Often mistakenly called 'imperforate hymen', it is very easily corrected. The key feature in all cases is a pelvic mass formed by the collected menses.

2. Minor endocrine disorder of control of the hypothalamic-pituitary-ovarian axis, in which there is failure of cyclicity but continuous basal ovarian follicular activity resulting in enough oestradiol to stimulate the oestrogen-responsive organs. There is an inherent, and life-long, defect of cycle initiation. Occasional spontaneous cycles do occur and are then normal and fertile. In such girls not only may the menarche be delayed but subsequent intermenstrual intervals are prolonged, sometimes to more than a year. The diagnostic feature is prompt ovulatory response to treatment with clomiphene, which simply initiates a cycle by inhibiting negative feedback on gonadotrophin secretion (see Chapter 11).

3. Testicular feminization, rarely (*see* Male Pseudohermaphroditism *above*). The key features are normal development of the breasts and female body shape, absent androgenic features (axillary and pubic hair), absent or short vagina, and absent uterus. The testicles may be intra-abdominal or may be palpable in the inguinal or labial region. The risk of malignant neoplasia (dysgerminoma) requires orchidectomy after puberty, with subsequent oestrogen replacement.

Precocious Puberty
This is defined as breast development commencing at or before 7 years of age, and menarche at or before 9 years. Pregnancy has been recorded in a 5-year-old (*see Guinness Book of Records*!). Precocious puberty is sometimes due to an endocrine-secreting tumour (and is then called precocious

pseudopuberty) of the ovaries or adrenal cortex, even rarely of the hypo-thalamus or pituitary. Most commonly precocious puberty merely represents one extreme of normal, since by definition the normal range includes only 95 per cent of the 'normal' population. In very young girls it presents a desperate problem – epiphyseal closure leads to gross limitation of height, and libido and aggression can cause major behavioural problems.

A tumour must always be sought, sometimes by laparotomy. In the other ('true') cases the recent development of the antigonadotrophic agent, danazol, offers new hope of delaying the progress of this serious disability.

THE MENOPAUSE

This means the cessation of menstrual periods and occurs on average at 51 years (normal range 44–58 years). 'The climacteric' is generally used to denote the perimenopausal years when most symptoms related to the menopause occur – mainly after the menopause but not infrequently before. The periods may stop suddenly or the cycle may first gradually lengthen, so that in practice recognition of the menopause requires 6 months' amenorrhoea. Even so, ovarian follicular activity and menstruation sometimes occur up to a year after the apparent menopause and can be confused with more worrying causes of postmenopausal bleeding (see Chapter 5). The age of menopause is unrelated to the age of menarche or to parity.

Mechanism
Ovarian failure is the primary event of the menopause, but the ovary is not completely depleted of primordial follicles. A minimum number of fol-licles seems to be required for a normal cycle to occur but little is known of the mechanism of control. Follicular control of gonadotrophin secretion by negative feedback involves not only oestradiol and progesterone but also inhibin. Thus the ovarian cycles leading up to the menopause are often infertile, despite apparently adequate steroid production, and are often associated with already high gonadotrophin levels, particularly FSH, typical of after the menopause (serum FSH >40 i.u./litre). These changes probably explain why menstrual disturbances are so common the last few years before the menopause.

After the menopause hypothalamic-pituitary changes also occur over many years resulting in gradual decline in gonadotrophin levels. There is a concomitant gradual decline in oestrogen levels, after the abrupt fall that occurs at the menopause. Oestrogen levels are very variable between individual women. Not only is there still some oestradiol secretion by the ovary, but also oestrone is produced by peripheral conversion in fat tissue from adrenocortical and ovarian androgen precursors (particularly androstenedione). Thus fat women after the menopause are better oestrogenized than thin women, but they are also at greater risk of endometrial carcinoma.

Effect and Complications

After the menopause, oestrogen deficiency leads to atrophy of the genital tract and lower urethra, atrophy of the breasts and skin, loss of the typically feminine body fat distribution, and gradual osteoporosis which eventually results in the stoop and loss of height typical of very old age with susceptibility to fractures.

Hot flushes are bouts of sometimes severe cutaneous vasodilatation, often with sweating, extending over the upper body. Their cause is uncertain but they can be largely suppressed by oestrogens or progestogens.

Genital atrophy can lead to vulvovaginal dryness, irritation and dyspareunia, excoriation and bleeding, and sometimes discharge due to secondary bacterial infection – all aspects of so-called atrophic vulvovaginitis (sometimes improperly named 'senile').

Various urinary symptoms are often due to lower urethral atrophy and stenosis associated with vulval atrophy.

Psychological disorders, particularly depression, insomnia and lack of libido, often occur after the menopause and can be severe. They may be mainly due to reaction to circumstances – loss of fertility, attractiveness (real or imagined), grown-up children – but may colour all the other symptoms occurring at this time, and any other coincidental illness too.

Treatment

Hot flushes and atrophic vulvovaginitis are the only disorders that really respond to oestrogen administration (in the latter case local application is effective), although even in these cases there is also a strong placebo effect. Urinary symptoms may respond to local oestrogen therapy but may also require surgical dilatation of the urethra. Nearly all other symptoms mainly require a sympathetic ear and advice.

Osteoporosis can be prevented but not reversed by oestrogen therapy, which is an argument for life-long prophylaxis. However, this must be balanced against the risks of thromboembolism and other possible vascular disorders. Oestrogen treatment can also cause endometrial cancer, but this is probably avoidable by giving the oestrogen cyclically and in combination with progestogen. The optimum preparation, route, dose and cycle remain uncertain. At present, treatment is only clearly indicated for specific symptoms (*see above*) and should be given in the lowest effective dose. It is not usually needed permanently and should be stopped every few months to try without.

Premature Menopause

This is due to primary ovarian failure occurring before the age of 40 years after a previously normal and often fertile, although shortened, menstrual career. It can be distinguished from other specific causes of primary ovarian failure presenting with secondary amenorrhoea (*see* Chapter 10), such as ovarian autoantibodies or damage. Its cause is unknown but it must be due to excessive atresia of primordial follicles or deficiency of the original number.

Primary ovarian failure is an uncommon cause of secondary amenorrhoea. This symptom should always be investigated before the age of 40 years (*see* Chapter 10), and even after that age pregnancy should of course not be overlooked.

Further Reading

Dewhurst C. J. (ed.) (1974) *Paediatric and Adolescent Gynaecology. Clinics in Obstetrics and Gynaecology,* 1 (3). Eastbourne, Saunders.

Greenblatt R. B. and Studd J. W. W. (ed.) (1977) *The Menopause. Clinics in Obstetrics and Gynaecology,* 4 (1). Eastbourne, Saunders.

Marshall W. A. and Tanner J. M. (1974) Chapter on Puberty. In: Davis J. A. and Dobbing J. (ed.) *Scientific Foundations of Paediatrics.* London, Heinemann.

Chapter ten

Endocrine and Related Disorders

Amenorrhoea

Amenorrhoea, the absence of menstruation, occurs as a physiological event during pregnancy and, of course, before normal menarche and after the menopause.

Pathological amenorrhoea is defined as the failure to menstruate for at least 6 months during the normal reproductive years in the absence of pregnancy, i.e. between 16 years (the limit for delayed menarche) and 40 years (the limit for premature menopause). Some authors require 12 months' amenorrhoea for their definition, but any figure chosen is arbitrary and the diversity reflects the overlap between amenorrhoea and oligomenorrhoea (*see below*). It occurs in 1–2 per cent of all women of reproductive age.

Amenorrhoea can be classified as primary, which is defined as for delayed menarche, i.e. failure to menstruate by the age of 16 years or later; or secondary, when menstruation has previously occurred. This distinction is of little practical value since the causes overlap. For instance, a partial form of ovarian dysgenesis can occur which, despite almost typical 'streak' ovaries, can present with secondary amenorrhoea. The distinction can even be misleading because some girls describe having menstruated when that was clearly impossible, being the result of optimistic imagination or traumatic self-examination.

Amenorrhoea is only a symptom, not a diagnosis. It is the common presenting feature of a variety of distinct disorders. These are nearly always endocrine disorders (99 per cent) and only occasionally due to anatomical defects (1 per cent).

Anatomical Causes
These can be summarized:

1. congenital:
   intersex states (*see* Chapter 9)
   vaginal atresia or uterine absence

2. acquired:
    endometrial fibrosis
    cervical stenosis.

The congenital defects present of course with primary amenorrhoea, the acquired ones with secondary. Some intersex states are due, fundamentally, to endocrine disorder, e.g. congenital adrenal hyperplasia (*see* Chapter 9).

Endometrial fibrosis (leading to occlusion of the cavity) may be due to tuberculosis, or to traumatic curettage, done usually after abortion or childbirth (Asherman's syndrome). Cervical stenosis may also be due to surgery, particularly cautery or conization.

Endocrine Causes

These can be classified as in Table 10.1, which also shows how commonly each condition is seen in practice, its underlying causes and diagnostic features.

Primary Hypothalamic or Pituitary Failure

Primary hypothalamic failure (*see* Chapter 9 on Delayed Puberty) should theoretically be demonstrable by gonadotrophin releasing hormone deficiency, but since that cannot be measured the disorder can only be recognized by the consequent gonadotrophin deficiency, as for primary pituitary failure. The gonadotrophin deficiency has to be demonstrated by failure to respond to an intravenous injection of releasing hormone. In these conditions ovulation can be induced by gonadotrophin therapy. (This treatment requires careful monitoring of ovarian oestrogen production to avoid hyperstimulation, which can result in large ovarian cysts and massive peritoneal effusion, or high-multiple pregnancy.) If pregnancy is not desired, oestrogen replacement therapy may be needed if there are symptoms due to deficiency, including secondary sexual immaturity.

Primary Ovarian Failure

Whatever the cause, this is permanent and irreversible. It may present with primary or secondary amenorrhoea, depending on the cause. As in the postmenopausal woman there is oestrogen deficiency and consequent high gonadotrophin levels, and some patients are troubled by hot flushes and atrophic vaginitis. High serum FSH (>40 i.u./litre) is the diagnostic feature rather than LH which may be raised in other disorders like the polycystic ovary syndrome. There is no treatment except oestrogen replacement for symptomatic deficiency. The finality of the diagnosis, especially its implication for future fertility, makes its confirmation by visualization and perhaps biopsy of the ovaries advisable. This is partly because of an uncommon variant called 'resistant ovaries' which may correct spon-

Table 10.1.   Endocrine disorders causing amenorrhoea and their underlying conditions, relative incidence, diagnostic features and consequent oestrogen state

Cause	Percentage	Diagnostic feature	Oestrogen state
1. Primary failure of the hypothalamic– pituitary–ovarian axis			
a Primary hypothalamic failure	1	LH, FSH deficiency	Deficient
Kallman' syndrome (permanent)			
Delayed puberty (temporary)			
b Primary pituitary failure	1		
Tumour			
Ablation			
Necrosis (Sheehan's syndrome)			
c Primary ovarian failure	10	Serum FSH high	Deficient
Dysgenesis			
Steroid enzyme defect			
Damage (surgery, irradiation)			
Autoantibodies			
Premature menopause			
2. Other discrete/measurable disorders			
a Hyperprolactinaemia	20	Serum prolactin high	Deficient
Pituitary tumours (8 per cent*)			
Primary hypothyroidism			
Drugs			
b Polycystic ovary syndrome	5	Hirsutism	Normal or high
c Other ? causes	2		
Thyroid disorders			
Diabetes mellitus			
Addison's disease			
3. 'Hypothalamic' disorders		Exclusion of all above disorders	
a Feedback disorders	45	– and anovulatory response to clomiphene	Deficient
Psychological disorder especially with weight loss			
b Cycle initiation defect	15	– and ovulatory response to clomiphene	Normal

*i.e. 8 per cent of all cases of amenorrhoea.

taneously (although attempts to induce ovulation are fruitless). 'Resistant ovaries' are characterized by plentiful but sometimes bizarre follicles associated with adequate oestrogen production (i.e. adequate to produce normal secondary changes) as well as high FSH levels. There is presumably a deficiency of inhibin, but this cannot yet be measured.

Hyperprolactinaemia
The existence of prolactin in humans and its important role in both normal and abnormal reproductive function has only emerged in the last

10 years when it could be assayed. Excess prolactin blocks the gonadal response to gonadotrophins, and also interferes with the control of gonadotrophin secretion, although normal amounts are present in the pituitary. Thus it causes secondary ovarian failure and consequent oestrogen deficiency, but gonadotrophin levels are not raised.

Of all the trophic hormones of the anterior pituitary only prolactin is controlled mainly by inhibition from the hypothalamus; the others are controlled mainly by release. Thus tumours compressing the hypothalamus or pituitary stalk cause panhypopituitarism but hyperprolactinaemia. Since the prolactin inhibiting factor from the hypothalamus is probably dopamine, many drugs with a dopamine-antagonistic action (and having a wide range of therapeutic uses) can cause hyperprolactinaemia and thus amenorrhoea. Also, since prolactin release can be stimulated by large amounts of thyrotrophin releasing hormone, primary thyroid failure can present with secondary hyperprolactinaemia and amenorrhoea. However, a pituitary chromophobe adenoma secreting prolactin is the commonest demonstrable cause of hyperprolactinaemia. At one time thought to be 'functionless', this tumour is now called a prolactinoma. It is found in about 40 per cent of cases of hyperprolactinaemia if carefully sought: tomography of the pituitary fossa is essential. In many of the other cases there may be a micro-tumour present which is not demonstrable radio-logically. It is a benign tumour which may grow very little in a whole life-time, but may threaten sight and life by growing rapidly upwards to compress the optic tracts or laterally into the cavernous sinus to cause thrombosis or bleeding.

Since prolactin is the stimulus for normal lactation, galactorrhoea (see later) is a common (but unreliable) symptom of hyperprolactinaemia. This association, with other unimportant features, has received various eponymous descriptions (e.g. the Chiari—Frommel and Forbes—Albright syndromes) in older books, but these terms are obsolete now that the essential feature, hyperprolactinaemia, has been recognized.

TREATMENT

Except when there is a large tumour, prolactin secretion can be suppressed very easily, using the dopamine agonist, bromocriptine, which is a synthetic ergot alkaloid. Prolactin levels fall quickly to normal, and the ovaries commence function almost immediately. The treatment is so effective and simple that it is easy to overlook the potential danger from a tumour if pregnancy ensues. The large amounts of placental oestrogens in pregnancy stimulate maternal prolactin secretion causing the normal pituitary to double in size, and a tumour may similarly undergo expansion with particular risk to the optic tracts. If pregnancy is desired a tumour may need to be treated first, and during pregnancy visual field perimetry should be done repeatedly. Small tumours can now be removed selectively via a trans-sphenoidal approach; large tumours require a transfrontal approach. Radiotherapy by beam or implants is an alternative. If amenorrhoea persists after treatment of a tumour it is usually due to incomplete treatment and consequent persistent hyperprolactinaemia (albeit at a lower level). Less often it is due to hypopituitarism.

Polycystic Ovary Syndrome

This poorly understood disorder is due to excessive androgen production by the ovaries and/or adrenal cortex, which interferes with ovarian follicular ripening. A large number of follicles develop abnormally, each to only about 5 mm diameter, crowded around the whole ovarian cortex and often enlarging the ovary generally. Occasionally the cause is an androgenic tumour of the ovary (of which there are various types: hilar-cell tumour, adrenal-like tumour and arrhenoblastoma) or of the adrenal cortex.

The typical features are (1) the appearance of the ovaries (if in practice they are looked at) and (2) hirsutism. Other common features are: (3) obesity, this in turn causing (4) excessive oestrogen production (by subcutaneous conversion of androgen precursors), (5) high LH levels, possibly stimulated by positive feedback of oestrogens on the hypothalamus; in turn the high LH and disproportionately low FSH levels possibly combine to induce abnormal ovarian follicular development and excess androgen production; (6) reduction in circulating levels of sex hormone binding globulin (SHBG) induced by excess testosterone, thus increasing the unbound (i.e. active) fraction of circulating testosterone; in turn, the increased availability of testosterone induces (7) greater enzymic metabolism of testosterone in hair follicles. It can thus be seen that whatever may be the origin of the disorder, a 'vicious circle' develops in which hyperandrogenism is self-promoting.

It is difficult to measure excess androgen production using routine laboratory methods. Circulating concentrations of total testosterone are often not elevated, but hide the increase in the unbound fraction. The best guide is the presence of hirsutism (see later). It is important always to enquire about it because at first sight one can be deceived by the effect of cosmetic treatment. When apparent, it is essential to distinguish true hirsutism from the constitutional form found in women from naturally hairy and dark-complexioned families. The latter will not, of course, respond to hormone therapy.

The other important clinical distinction to be made is of an androgenic tumour. The best guides are signs of virilism in addition to hirsutism, particularly clitoral enlargement, and the finding of very high circulating levels of testosterone. In that case the ovaries need to be split open to seek an often small hilar tumour, and the adrenal veins catheterized to measure testosterone outflow.

There is an associated risk of endometrial carcinoma because of the prolonged stimulation with oestrogen unopposed by progestogen without shedding of the endometrium. Not all women with the polycystic ovary syndrome have amenorrhoea, however; a few menstruate more or less normally, although they seldom ovulate.

TREATMENT

A tumour should be excised. In the much more common functional disorder, treatment may be aimed at hirsutism, infertility or both, and there is also the need to induce regular menstruation to protect against endometrial carcinoma. Hirsutism may be treated by combined oestrogen/ progestogen oral contraception (to induce SHBG and so 'mop up' excess unbound testosterone) and by the antiandrogen, cyproterone acetate (see section on Hirsutism). Normal follicular maturation (and consequent ovulation) can usually be induced by the antioestrogen, clomiphene (by inhibiting negative feedback resulting in increased secretion of FSH); excision of a large wedge from each ovary is (somehow) also often effective, but its effect is temporary and it may lead to adhesions. Menstruation can be induced by a short course of progestogen (e.g. medroxyprogesterone acetate 5 mg daily for 5 days), and can be repeated regularly. Effective total therapy is sometimes achieved with glucocorticoids if the disorder is primarily adrenal. Finally, it is likely that obesity plays a key role in maintaining, if not initiating, the disorder, and dietary advice should be given to reduce weight to normal (in practice refer to *Fig.* 10.1).

Other Discrete Endocrine Disorders

Amenorrhoea is rarely found to be associated with thyroid disorders (1 per cent), diabetes mellitus or Addison's disease (<1 per cent), and their finding may be coincidental. Primary hypothyroidism is, however, a well-defined, if uncommon, cause of hyperprolactinaemia and consequent amenorrhoea. Symptoms of thyroid disorder should therefore always be sought.

Hypothalamic Disorders

The term implies disorder (not primary failure) of the hypothalamic control of the hypothalamic-pituitary-ovarian axis, not due to any demonstrable endocrine abnormality originating outside this axis. The majority of cases are due to 'environmental' influences, particularly psychological disorders and weight loss. Their mode of action on the hypothalamus is unknown, but the fact that they disturb the hypothalamus is shown by disorder of functions like body temperature control.

Hypothalamic disorder causing amenorrhoea is recognized in practice by exclusion of all the discrete disorders mentioned, i.e. by finding normal serum FSH, prolactin and thyroid hormone levels and absence of hirsutism. Hypothalamic disorders can be subclassified in endocrinological terms according to the response to a 5-day course of oral clomiphene as shown in Table 10.1. (Clomiphene stimulates follicular maturation by its antioestrogen action inhibiting normal negative feedback of oestrogen on gonadotrophin secretion.) This does not mean, however, that ovulation in response to clomiphene never occurs in patients with discrete disorders, although in fact of the latter only those with polycystic ovary disease usually do so and rarely patients with hyperprolactinaemia.

When amenorrhoea is due to weight loss and/or psychological disorder the reproductive disturbance is severe. It is characterized by disordered feedback control on gonadotrophin secretion with consequent oestrogen deficiency and failure to ovulate in response to clomiphene. Induction of ovulation in these cases may be achieved by psychological treatment but usually it is necessary to use gonadotrophin (Pergonal) injections. This requires great care to avoid ovarian hyperstimulation, which can be dangerous.

By contrast, the cycle initiation defect seems to be an inherent disorder, in some respects not unlike polycystic ovary disease. The patients appear normal in every way apart from their amenorrhoea; they are oestrogenized and demonstrate normal feedback mechanisms on gonadotrophin secretion by their ovulatory response to clomiphene. In fact spontaneous ovulatory cycles occur occasionally, and these patients sometimes find themselves unexpectedly pregnant.

Weight Loss and Psychological Disorders

Psychological disorder or stress is the commonest cause of amenorrhoea (Table 10.1) and accounts for its frequency in young women leaving home for the first time and starting institutional training. This is also commonly associated with weight loss, which may be the primary cause of the amenorrhoea. Another common cause of weight loss leading to amenorrhoea, usually in adolescence, is cosmetic dieting which gets out of control. A loss of more than 10 kg (1½ stones) seems to be the danger mark. Whatever the original cause or motive for dieting, it is important to appreciate that for some young women it becomes an obsession which can lead to anorexia nervosa.

Anorexia nervosa is misnamed because there is no loss of appetite. The girl (she is usually teenage) is obsessed with her size and starves herself but cannot of course admit it. In its chronic form anorexia nervosa is a life-long disorder with distinct psychological features still centred on obsession with weight control long after most of the original weight loss has been restored. It accounts for 10–15 per cent of all women complaining of amenorrhoea. Altogether, a history of weight loss with or without the distinct features of anorexia nervosa accounts for 25–30 per cent of women with amenorrhoea.

It is important to appreciate that the major weight loss usually occurred at the start of the amenorrhoea and much of the original loss has usually been regained. These patients are no longer extremely thin (although often

well below average weight – refer to *Fig.* 10.1 in practice). At first sight
they appear unremarkable – perhaps modishly slim and a little reserved
– and as a result their underlying condition is frequently missed. A careful
history of weight fluctuation and psychological factors should always be
taken in amenorrhoea. Much stress and unhappiness is likely to be un-
covered. Also, regaining the lost weight is a sure means of restoring
reproductive function, and far preferable to treatment with gonadotrophins
(Pergonal), which is otherwise required to induce ovulation when pregnancy is desired.

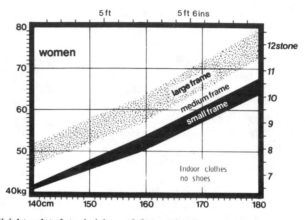

Fig. 10.1. Weight related to height and frame size in normal women. (Reproduced
from G. W. Thorpe (1974), *Medicine* (Series 1, No. 28, p. 1658) with kind permission
of the Editor.)

Obesity and Amenorrhoea

There are minor changes in the differential release of FSH and LH, and
there is increased adrenal cortisol and possibly androgen production, in
obese women compared with normal. However, there is no clear association
between amenorrhoea and obesity (unlike weight loss), except in the
polycystic ovary syndrome. It is thus unpredictable (in contrast to weight
restoration in the underweight) whether reduction of weight in obese
patients will restore menstruation, but it seems to be advisable anyway for
wider reasons.

Oral Contraception and Amenorrhoea

There is often a slight delay in resumption of menstruation after stopping
combined oestrogen–progestogen oral contraception. The average delay is
only a week and it seldom lasts 6 months. In the latter case the term
'post-pill amenorrhoea' is commonly used (in the UK and the USA, but
not continental Europe) to imply a causative association. However, there is
no strong evidence that this is so. The endocrine disorders found are the

same as in amenorrhoeic women who have not used oral contraception, suggesting that 'post-pill amenorrhoea' is not an entity, and the need for investigation (*see below*) should not be disregarded. The coincidental nature of the association is explained by the artificially induced menstruation which masks the underlying condition for the duration of the oral contraception.

Amenorrhoea occurring during oral contraception is less easily explained — it may be due to prompt return of ovarian oestrogen production in the pill-free interval, thus maintaining the endometrium — but can be disregarded. It is mainly only a nuisance, causing concern about possible pregnancy.

Investigation of Amenorrhoea

The basic investigations needed can be summarized as follows:

1. history:
   weight fluctuation
   psychological factors
   thyroid symptoms
   drug usuage
   hirsutism
   (hot flushes: unreliable guide to primary ovarian faulure but may need symptomatic relief)
   (galactorrhoea: unreliable guide to hyperprolactinaemia but may need symptomatic relief)
2. examination:
   hirsutism (and other signs of virilization)
   integrity of genital tract
   (oestrogen state of the genital tract: inessential diagnostic feature but may need symptomatic relief)
3. hormone measurements:
   FSH
   prolactin
   thyroid hormones (especially free thyroxine index)
4. lateral skull X-ray
5. clomiphene response (only when pregnancy is desired).

Treatment of Amenorrhoea

The treatment is of the cause (*see* Table 10.1) if possible. Patients with psychological causes or weight loss should be the most amenable but often are very resistant to any change in their behaviour. When pregnancy is desired, ovulation induction is usually achieved not by fundamental correction of the underlying cause but by temporarily getting around the reproductive disorder using, most commonly, clomiphene, bromocriptine or gonadotrophins as appropriate.

Alternatively, contraception may be needed. Since ovulation occurs sporadically in some disorders (e.g. polycystic ovary syndrome and cycle initiation defect), and other common disorders (due to psychological factors or weight loss) may resolve spontaneously, reliable methods should be used if contraception is needed. Since there is no strong evidence to implicate oral contraceptives as a cause of amenorrhoea they may be used as usual. Oestrogen preparations are, however, better avoided in hyperprolactinaemia for fear of stimulating the growth of any existing pituitary tumour.

Oligomenorrhoea

Oligomenorrhoea is defined as menstrual cycles prolonged to between 6 weeks and 6 months. At one end of the spectrum it overlaps with normal, the cycles being ovulatory but infrequent. At the other, it overlaps with amenorrhoea and shares all the same causes (Table 10.1) except primary failure of the components of the hypothalamic-pituitary-ovarian axis, which causes permanent amenorrhoea.

Oligomenorrhoeic cycles may be ovulatory or anovulatory, depending on the cause. It is not important in practice to make this distinction, only to investigate possibly serious underlying causes which may need treatment, particularly a prolactinoma, androgenic tumour, thyroid disorder or psychological disturbance. If infertility is an associated problem and discrete endocrine disorders can be excluded, it is easier to organize investigation of ovulation (which is difficult when cycles are long and irregular) in response to treatment with clomiphene. This shortens the cycle predictably and thereby also improves the chance of conception.

Hirsutism

Hirsutism is the occurrence of male sexual hair, namely (1) stout, pigmented ('terminal') hair on the face, upper pubic triangle and chest, and spreading laterally from the lower pubic triangle, on the thighs and in the nose and ears, (2) thin, unpigmented ('vellus') hairs replacing terminal hairs in the temporal and vertical areas of the scalp (i.e. male-pattern balding). In addition there is accentuation of ambosexual hair, i.e. terminal hair stimulated by low levels of androgens (from the adrenals and ovaries) in the axillae, pubic area, forearms and lower legs.

Hirsutism is only one feature of virilism, which includes clitoromegaly, deepening of the voice and muscular prominence. However, hirsutism without baldness is usually the only presenting feature of virilism. In the absence of these other features it can often be difficult to distinguish between 'true' and 'constitutional' hirsutism. True hirsutism is due to excessive androgens, whereas constitutional hirsutism is a normal feature of certain races and tribes. There is much overlap in the hairiness of normal women and men, particularly evident when comparing Southern European women with Mongoloid men. The majority of European women have terminal hair on the forearms and lower legs, and a quarter have it on the face, upper lip, upper pubic triangle or chest. Although in true hirsutism androgen levels in blood and urine are on average greater than normal, levels in individuals are often in the normal range. It now seems that increased unbound testosterone in serum is a reliable index in these cases but it is not so easily determined as total testosterone. Associated menstrual disorder and (if looked for) polycystic ovaries support a diagnosis of true hirsutism, whereas constitutional hirsutism is more likely in swarthy women with hirsute relatives.

The causes of true hirsutism and their investigation is as for the polycystic ovary syndrome (*see* section on Amenorrhoea).

Treatment
Although treatment is necessarily protracted and often unsuccessful, every effort should be made because hirsutism can be a distressing stigma. Success of treatment hinges on accurate diagnosis. An androgenic tumour should be excised, but it is rare. If hyperandrogenism originates in the adrenal cortex glucocorticoid treatment is effective. If ovarian disturbance is responsible it can be partly suppressed by combined oestrogen/ progestogen oral contraception. Often the cause is not distinct and then treatment is unreliable. In these cases an oral contraceptive is used in order to stimulate production of sex hormone binding globulin, so as to reduce the amount of circulating unbound testosterone. In addition, a newly available steroidal antiandrogen, cyproterone acetate, seems to be very effective by acting directly on the hair follicles. It needs to be used carefully because it is cumulative, and should be combined with an oral contraceptive because it is highly teratogenic for the fetus. If pregnancy occurs it should be terminated. In all cases treatment must be continued for 6–12 months before the hirsutism can be expected to diminish because of the length of the growth cycle of the hair follicle.

When treatment is unsuccessful, or in cases of constitutional hirsutism, the only recourse is to cosmetic measures. When electrolysis of hair follicles is skilfully done it is remarkably good, but it needs repeating and is moderately expensive, and so is usually confined to the face. The alternatives are shaving, depilatory creams, bleaching and cosmetic make-up.

Galactorrhoea

Galactorrhoea is inappropriate, i.e. non-puerperal, lactation. In the majority of cases it amounts to only a few milky drops on firm manipulation of the breast and nipple, but can occur spontaneously and require constant wearing of absorbent pads. It is usually bilateral.

There are two main causes, which account about equally for most cases – hyperprolactinaemia and mechanical stimulation of the breasts. The few remaining cases have no recognizable cause, although in some galactorrhoea occurs only during oral contraception. Galactorrhoea itself is probably not harmful, although it might be a nuisance, but may be important as a symptom of hyperprolactinaemia, which is often due to a pituitary tumour (see section on Amenorrhoea). Treatment should be aimed at the cause and bromocriptine should not be used indiscriminately. Since hyperprolactinaemia nearly always causes oligo- or amenorrhoea it can safely be assumed not to be the cause of galactorrhoea when menstruation is normal.

Physical stimulation is the usual cause of galactorrhoea persisting after breast-feeding in a woman with normal menstrual cycles. It is even possible in this way to induce lactation long after breast-feeding (and even in nulliparous women), sufficient to feed another baby — hence the wet-nurses of old. The mechanism is by neuroendocrine reflex secretion of prolactin. The stimulation is often done out of curiosity 'to see if there is still any milk there', in which case avoidance is easy and effective. However, if the stimulation is sexual it may be hard to give up and there seems no need to insist on it, but temporary avoidance is worth trying because it may be permanently effective.

Galactorrhoea during combined oestrogen–progestogen contraception is also likely to be due to physical stimulation or hyperprolactinaemia. In the latter case, however, the expected clue of amenorrhoea will be masked by the artificially induced bleeds. If galactorrhoea does not stop soon after avoidance of physical stimulation it will be necessary to determine the serum prolactin concentration.

Galactorrhoea occurring only during oral contraception and not other-wise is difficult to explain. This is partly because the hormonal control of breast development and lactation (see Chapter 12) is remarkably complicated, involving not only oestrogens, progesterone and prolactin but also growth hormone, cortisol and thyroid hormones. The oestrogen–progestogen contraceptive pill certainly increases prolactin secretion, but not to abnormal levels. In addition to acting directly on the breast it also modifies the effect of other hormones by increasing the circulating amounts of their binding proteins. There seems no need to stop oral contraception just because of galactorrhoea.

Further Reading
Hull M. G. R. (1980) Amenorrhoea: advances in practice. *Hospital Update* 6, 219.
Hull M. G. R. (1979) Dietary restriction and amenorrhoea. *J. Mat. Child Health* 4, 104.
Mishell D. R. and Davajan V. (1979) *Reproductive Endocrinology, Infertility and Contraception.* Philadelphia, Davis.
Yen S. S. C. and Jaffe R. B. (1978) *Reproductive Endocrinology.* Philadelphia, Saunders.

Chapter eleven

Infertility and Early Pregnancy Wastage

Infertility is a common problem, and may indeed be the most common complaint or potential complaint of the young adult population. Well over 10 per cent of women in all Western countries are childless, and probably at least 10 per cent of couples are involuntarily infertile. Some will accept and adapt to the childless state without untoward effects, but for many it produces emotional problems of considerable proportions. This can be a very rewarding area for the interested gynaecologist or general practitioner, and the necessary skills and background knowledge are not difficult to acquire. On the other hand, disinterested or inaccurate advice is worse than useless.

The average time for normal couples to take to get pregnant is 6 cycles, and 10 per cent take longer than one year. However, it is unreasonable to withhold investigations from couples who are concerned about not having got pregnant even if they have been trying for less than a year. Very often there is no single, clear factor accounting for the couple's infertility, but a number of suboptimal features which together make it less likely that the couple will conceive in any one cycle and extend their time to achieve a pregnancy. The situation may be aggravated by anxiety adversely affecting ovarian function. The considerable number of pregnancies that occur during the course of investigations (as opposed to treatment) are no doubt partly produced by the reassurance that would normally accompany investigations.

Causes of Infertility

1. Defective ovulation (anovular cycles, poor luteal phase, oligomenorrhoea, amenorrhoea) – 25 per cent.
2. Defective semen (oligospermia and azoospermia) – 25 per cent.
3. Tubal blockage – 15 per cent.
4. Other gynaecological abnormalities (fibroids, endometriosis, etc.) – 7 per cent.
5. Immunity problems (female sperm antibodies or male auto-antibodies) – 3 per cent.

6. Normal couples with no abnormality found after full investigations — 20 per cent.
7. Other problems. Endometrial TB used to account for 5 per cent of infertility but is now extremely rare in this country. Failure to consummate marriage may occasionally be seen, particularly in general practice, and the complaint of infertility is sometimes a more acceptable way for the patient to seek help with sexual problems.
8. Other medical disorders. Most serious medical disorders, and particularly endocrine dysfunction, can produce infertility but in ·practice they are rarely seen in infertility clinics. A modest degree of clinical alertness is usually sufficient to pick up such cases, and there is no place for screening all patients for general endocrine disease in the absence of clinical suspicion.

Investigations

General Principles

It is generally more effective and certainly kinder to the couple to investigate them as a couple rather than as individuals in two separate clinics, where conflicting advice may be given or important mutual problems such as sperm—cervical mucus incompatiblilty may be overlooked. It is also usually advisable to look at a full range of investigations, even if a clear cause for infertility is found early in the investigations; it is, for instance, very common to find defective ovulation in the wife when the husband has azoospermia or oligospermia. However, it is probably unreasonable to proceed to a test for tubal patency such as laparoscopy in cases of azoospermia where it is clear that the wife has not had an opportunity to demonstrate her fertility. It is important to have a clear aim in mind for any investigation and not simply to repeat investigations or carry on with basal temperature recording as a time-wasting manoeuvre. There are five important areas to check as follows:

Ovulation

The occurrence of ovulation and the length of the luteal phase can be checked by basal temperature recording. Examples of a normal ovulatory cycle, an anovular cycle and a short luteal phase are shown in *Fig.* 11.1. The basal temperature can be taken orally but in order to make this reliable it is essential that the woman takes her temperature in bed in the morning before doing anything else. As long as a little time is spent explaining the basic principles of temperature recording the majority of patients will produce satisfactory records. The most likely time for ovulation is the last day before the temperature rise but this is not precise. Research has shown that the actual day of ovulation may be 3 days in either direction of this low point in the temperature chart so that no useful purpose is served by asking the couple to confine intercourse to that day. The elevated portion of the temperature chart should last at least 12

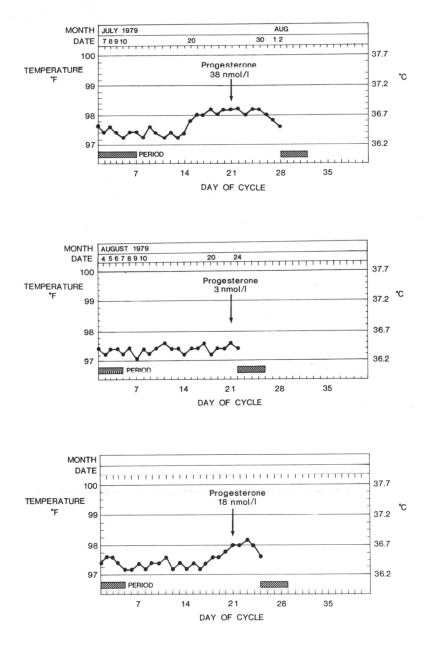

Fig. 11.1. Basal temperature records for a normal ovulatory cycle (top), an anovular cycle (centre) and a cycle with a short luteal phase (bottom).

days to give a reasonable chance of pregnancy, and anything less should be considered as a short luteal phase. There is little point in continuing with temperature charts for more than 3 months unless they are being used as an aid to check on the efficacy of induction of ovulation or as an aid to timing insemination.

Sperm Production, Delivery and Compatibility

The initial test of choice is a postcoital test, although experience and a certain amount of special equipment is needed for this to be satisfactory. For the postcoital test, cervical mucus is taken with some form of syringe at about the time of ovulation (day 13 or 14 of a 28-day cycle) with the couple having had intercourse between 6 and 24 hours previously, i.e. the night before. This mucus can then be examined under a simple light microscope and the numbers of sperms and their motility recorded. If large numbers of motile sperms are present (i.e. 30 or more per low power field) the husband is producing a satisfactory number of sperms, which are being ejaculated in the right place and are not suffering from any immunity problems. If sperms are present but all dead, or if there are no sperms or very few sperms, further investigation is needed. An alternative investigation is a semen analysis. This provides more precise information about the number of sperms produced but a less valuable indication of their quality and no information concerning their compatibility with the cervical mucus. In many cases both tests will be done, but although a good postcoital test avoids the need for semen analysis the reverse is not true. A normal semen analysis is usually taken as showing a volume of 2 ml or more, a sperm density of 40 million per ml or more, motility at 1 hour of over 40 per cent and sperm abnormality rate of less than 30 per cent. These figures, however, are arbitrary, particularly the sperm density figure, and fertile men may frequently be found with sperm densities well below 40 million per ml. There is, furthermore, great variation in an individual semen analysis, and consecutive sperm counts may vary by a factor of 10 or more. It is therefore unwise to give a firm opinion on the basis of a single semen analysis. Minor illnesses, particularly pyrexial illnesses, and also stress may adversely affect sperm counts for many months afterwards. After an attack of influenza, for instance, one can expect a drastically reduced sperm count for 6 months, followed by eventual recovery.

In the presence of a poor postcoital test and a normal semen analysis a mucus penetration test should be performed. A small portion of ovulatory cervical mucus and a drop of semen are placed next to each other on a slide and covered with a cover slip so that they coalesce and produce a vertical interface. The progress of the sperms can then be watched microscopically and agglutination, failure of invasion or immobilization of the sperms in the mucus can be detected. Autoantibodies are particularly associated with agglutination and failure of penetration. Female sperm antibodies are usually associated with normal penetration of the mucus together with marked sperm immobilization after 10 minutes.

Hormonal Function and Confirmation of Ovulation
The best indication of hormonal adequacy of the cycle is to measure progesterone in the mid-luteal phase, that is day 21 of a 28-day cycle. The normal values of serum progesterone at this stage of the cycle will be 30–60 nmol/l (10–20 ng/ml), but individual laboratory normals vary slightly. Luteal function depends closely on follicular function, and a good luteal phase is only seen with an adequate follicular phase. Conversely, the best treatment for an inadequate luteal phase is clomiphene given in early follicular phase. There is really no need or any point in other hormonal investigation, except for serum prolactin estimations in cases of persistently poor luteal function not responding to clomiphene. If serum progesterone estimations are not available, some idea of luteal function can be obtained by endometrial biopsy, but this is no longer generally used.

Tubal Patency and Normality of Reproductive Organs
The initial clinical examination should rule out gross pelvic abnormalities, but there are a number of factors such as peritubal adhesions, blocked Fallopian tubes, uterine fibroids and endometriosis which may escape the most skilled clinical examination. It has been shown that the most effective way of picking up such abnormalities is to do a laparoscopy, hydrotubation and dilatation and curettage, with curettings being sent for histology and culture for TB. Alternative means of demonstrating tubal patency are hysterosalpingography (X-rays taken after intrauterine injection of radio-opaque dye) and tubal insufflation (blowing carbon dioxide or nitrous oxide through the uterus and tubes with a special apparatus which produces a limited flow and pressure of gas). These two methods are less invasive but less efficient at picking up all pathology. This is particularly true of tubal insufflation and there is probably now no place for this in the routine investigation of infertility. The choice of laparoscopy or hysterosalpingography will depend on the facilities available within the locality. False negative tubal patency tests are possible with all these methods, and it is usually desirable to confirm a diagnosis of tubal blockage with another test before embarking on surgery. A hysterosalpingogram not only confirms a laparoscopic diagnosis of tubal blockage but also adds useful information about the extent of any tubal damage.

Further Investigation of the Oligo- Azoospermic Man
If semen analysis reveals azoospermia or significant oligospermia the husband should be further investigated. Enquiries are made into his general health and any history of infection, trauma or surgery to the genital area. Examination should include a general assessment of hair growth and other signs of virilization together with detailed assessment of the genitalia,

noting the size and consistency of each testicle, epididymis, and vas, examining the penis and also making a search for varicocoeles with the patient standing. If the man is not fully virilized or if there has been recent loss of libido or onset of impotence, gonadotrophin, testosterone and prolactin levels should be measured. If any of the stigmata of Klinefelter's syndrome are present, chromosome studies should be undertaken. Otherwise consideration may be given to a testicular biopsy. This may reveal total lack of germ cells or normal spermatogenesis (with blockage or agenesis of the vas or epididymis), failure of maturation or sloughing of the germinal epithelium. The latter findings are potentially treatable but unfortunately make up a small minority of cases. In men with testes of markedly reduced size but who are otherwise well androgenized the chances of finding a remediable lesion are negligible, and a testicular biopsy is probably not justified.

Treatment

Ovulatory Problems

Most forms of ovulatory failure and poor luteal phase should be treated in the first instance with clomiphene, starting with a dose of 50 mg daily from day 1 to day 5 of the cycle, increasing the dose as necessary up to a maximum of 200 mg a day for 5 days. Most women who are menstruating will respond to this, although only a minority of amenorrhoeic women will. The effectiveness of treatment should be checked by measuring serum progesterone in the mid-luteal phase and by checking that postcoital tests are satisfactory. If there is no response to clomiphene a serum prolactin should be ordered and, if it is not elevated, gonadotrophin treatment may be necessary. Gonadotrophin treatment is extremely expensive and potentially hazardous and is confined to specialist units. Overdosage may result in hyperstimulation of the ovaries with massive cyst formation, the possibility of high multiple pregnancy or even death of the patient. Hyperprolactinaemia is treated with bromocriptine (*see* Chapter 10).

Sperm Problems

The treatment of oligospermia is disappointing. Clomiphene 50 mg daily or mesterolone 25 mg t.d.s. may produce a modest elevation in sperm count, rarely by more than a factor of 10. Wearing loose underpants and avoiding long, hot baths may also produce similar improvements in sperm counts. There is probably no effective treatment for high abnormality rates. Low motility is sometimes due to chronic prostatitis and may respond to antibiotic treatment. If a varicocoele is present then ligation of the offending veins sometimes produces quite a striking improvement in the semen picture.

The treatment of azoospermia depends entirely on the underlying cause and prior investigation is essential. Blockage of the vas may be circumvented by an epididymovasostomy but the subsequent pregnancy rate is very low. Azoospermia associated with sloughing of the genital epithelium may be treated with methyltestosterone 15 mg daily sublingually for 3 months. Maturation arrest may respond to gonadotrophin treatment, but this again is confined to specialist units. Failing these relatively rare treatable situations, the only other therapeutic possibility is artificial insemination with donor semen (AID), which is available in most developed countries now. Alternatively, of course, the couple may consider adoption, but this is difficult in most parts of the world.

Sperm Antibodies
All forms of treatment of sperm autoantibodies have proved unsuccessful. For female sperm antibodies occasional success has been reported with the use of a sheath to avoid physical contact with semen over the course of 2 or 3 months followed by intercourse at the time of ovulation. Some success has also been claimed for intrauterine insemination of fresh semen at the time of ovulation (by-passing the cervical mucus which is the main site of sperm antibody production).

Tubal Problems
When a definitive diagnosis of tubal occlusion or peritubal adhesions has been made by laparoscopy or hysterosalpingography (or preferably both), tubal surgery may be considered, but the results are very bad: few hospitals have overall pregnancy rates following tubal surgery of more than 20 per cent and most are probably below this figure. The couple should be made aware of this gloomy prognosis before arrangements are made for surgery, but in practice most patients still welcome operation. The main operations are as follows:

Salpingostomy
This operation may be performed to relieve fimbrial blockage of the tubes. The end of the tube is either teased open or removed and the cut edge is usually turned back over the Fallopian tube as a cuff and sutured there. The pregnancy rate is poor and particularly so if tubes are diseased or distorted as hydrosalpinges.

Tubal Implantation
This operation may be performed for blockage of the inner portion of the tube. The diseased part is excised and the patent outer part of the tube is then implanted and fixed in the cornu of the uterus. The outlook is somewhat better than for salpingostomy but still probably does not exceed 20 per cent.

Tubal Reanastomosis
This operation is used to reverse sterilization operations. The obliterated part of the tube can be excised and an anastomosis performed over a

simple nylon splint. The pregnancy rate may be over 50 per cent if the tube is healthy and a very small portion of tube was removed at the original operation.

Salpingolysis
This involves simple division and removal of adhesions in and around the tube and ovary. Sheet adhesions between the fimbrial end of the tube and the ovary can totally interfere with normal mechanisms of egg capture, and if the tube is otherwise healthy the pregnancy rate can be quite high following this form of operation, but it is very much related to the extent and density of the adhesions.

Fibroids
Myomectomy may be performed but is only likely to be helpful if the fibroid impinges on the uterine cavity. Pregnancy rates following myomectomy are unlikely to exceed 50 per cent, and small fibroids that are not impinging on the cavity are probably best ignored.

Endometriosis
Endometriosis is a potent cause of infertility and may be treated either surgically or with hormones (*see* Chapter 3).

General Prognosis
About 50 per cent of all patients who have infertility investigations and treatment can be expected to achieve a pregnancy eventually. The pregnancy rate of treated patients exceeds that of untreated patients but not by a very large margin. In general the pregnancy rate is lower the longer the patient has been infertile, but there are exceptions to this rule, and the individual diagnosis provides a much surer means of predicting the outcome. Some infertility factors will also affect the course of the subsequent pregnancy, but in general the outcome of pregnancies of previously infertile women is not appreciably worse than average. Factors which should be closely watched are the possibility of ovulation induction producing high multiple pregnancy and leading to abortion, tubal surgery being associated with a high incidence of ectopic pregnancy, myomectomy or surgery for uterine abnormalities leading to the possibility of malpresentations or uterine scar rupture and the need to consider elective Caesarean section.

Early Pregnancy Wastage
First Trimester Abortion
About 1 in 7 of all pregnancies abort at this stage of pregnancy and the vast majority of those that do so are abnormal. In most cases there is no recurrent aetiological factor and the outlook for the subsequent pregnancy is not appreciably worse than average after one, two or even three

spontaneous abortions. Very occasionally there is a recurrent factor, and it is usual to investigate women who have had three spontaneous abortions.

Threatened Abortion
A threatened abortion is diagnosed when there is any bleeding from the genital tract before the twenty-eighth week of pregnancy and as long as no products of conception have been passed and the cervix remains undilated. Three out of four threatened abortions settle down, and when this happens there is no increased risk of fetal abnormality. The remainder abort and the abortion rate is not materially affected by any treatment. It is traditional to confine patients with threatened abortion to bed until a few days after the bleeding has stopped, and to rest and to avoid intercourse for at least 2 weeks. There is no evidence that any of these measures has any effect other than a psychological one. There is also no evidence that hormones are of any help in the treatment of threatened abortion (or recurrent abortion) and as there are a number of known adverse effects of steroid hormones given in early pregnancy they should not be used even for their psycho-therapeutic effects. Human placental lactogen and progesterone estimations may give some indication of prognosis, but misleading results are common, and skilled ultrasound examination of the uterus probably provides the best prognostic indicator.

Inevitable Abortion
An abortion becomes inevitable when the cervix dilates significantly or products of conception are passed. Most inevitable abortions are accompanied by a considerable amount of vaginal bleeding and low abdominal pain. Before 14 weeks it is usual for the placenta to be expelled incompletely and the risk of continued bleeding or uterine infection means that such cases are best admitted to hospital for evacuation of the uterus. The bleeding in incomplete abortions can occasionally be severe and necessitate a Flying Squad call to transfuse the patient before admission to hospital. Blood loss is usually controlled at least in part by ergometrine 0·5 mg i.m. or i.v. When the patient is seen a day or two after an abortion, signs that suggest it was incomplete are continued vaginal blood loss, a patulous cervix and a slightly bulky and tender uterus.

Complete Abortion
Following complete abortion there should be no appreciable vaginal blood loss, only a slight reddish discharge. The uterus is not tender and fairly rapidly returns to normal size. The cervix should be closed. Complete abortion needs no further treatment, but if there is any doubt at all it is better to perform an evacuation.

Septic Abortion
An incomplete abortion may occasionally become infected with organisms from the vagina or bowel and this is particularly likely if the abortion has

been procured illegally. The infection may spread from the uterine cavity to the parametrium and to the tubes and thence to the pelvic peritoneum. Death from generalized peritonitis, septicaemia or renal failure may result. Cases of septic abortion must be admitted urgently to hospital and treated with high-dose antibiotics, blood transfusion and general supportive measures and early evacuation of the septic products. There is a danger of long-term tubal blockage and sterility.

Recurrent Abortion

Recurrent abortion may be caused by the following:

chromosome abnormalities in either parent (such as translocations);
uterine abnormalities;
serious chronic illness, such as renal disease or syphilis;
incompetent cervix (although this usually produces middle trimester abortion);
mistaken diagnosis where the woman definitely wants to be pregnant and is having delayed periods.

In practice these factors only account for a few per cent of recurrent abortion when the woman has had three previous abortions. Nevertheless, in such cases it is usual to perform chromosomal investigations of the couple and to have a hysterosalpingogram to exclude congenital uterine abnormalities and intrauterine fibroids. When recurrent causes have been excluded the mainstay of treatment for recurrent first trimester abortion is tender loving care. However, such patients are often admitted to hospital for prolonged rest, although it is doubtful whether this is necessary or more effective than rest at home.

Second Trimester Abortion

The causes of middle trimester abortion are as follows:

uterine abnormalities;
cervical incompetence;
fetal abnormality;
intrauterine death of the fetus;
high multiple pregnancy;
maternal ill health.

There is a strong tendency for middle trimester abortion to be recurrent and all cases should be investigated after the first loss. If at all possible the fetus and placenta should be examined by a pathologist at the time of abortion, and if these are normal a hysterosalpingogram is advisable. Abnormalities such as a bicornuate uterus may sometimes be corrected surgically with subsequent pregnancies going to term. An incompetent cervix is treated by the insertion of a Shirodkar suture (*see* Chapter 13).

Hydatidiform Mole

Hydatidiform mole (already described fully in Chapter 6) may present as a threatened or incomplete abortion in either first or second trimester. It is very often associated with recurrent bleeding, and also with excessive uterine size and hyperemesis. In such circumstances the diagnosis of hydatidiform mole must be considered and either an ultrasound scan or an HCG estimation should be arranged to exclude it. When the products passed at the time of abortion include any vesicles they should be sent for histological examination, as careful follow-up of all cases of hydatidiform mole is important in order to minimize the risk of subsequent choriocarcinoma.

Ectopic Pregnancy

In about 1 in 500 pregnancies (in this country) an ovum may develop in a site other than the uterus, most commonly in the Fallopian tube but occasionally in the ovary, the uterine cavity or the pelvic peritoneum. The incidence varies around the world, principally in relation to the occurrence of pelvic inflammatory disease, although there is also an increased risk of ectopic pregnancy after tubal surgery, and with the use of intrauterine contraceptive devices or progestogen-only pills.

Clinical Features of Tubal Ectopic Pregnancies

The clinical picture depends on whether the ovum has implanted in the narrow part of the Fallopian tube (the isthmus) or in the wider outer portion (the ampulla). The lumen of the isthmus is 1 mm or less and the developing conceptus rapidly erodes its way through the tubal wall, presenting the features of a ruptured ectopic pregnancy:

1. Onset of symptoms around the time of first missed period.
2. Severe pain in pelvis and lower abdomen, and sometimes shoulder tips (diaphragmatic irritation).
3. Collapse – due to intraperitoneal haemorrhage, sometimes progressing rapidly to the death of the patient.
4. Slight dark red vaginal loss.
5. Marked tenderness on vaginal examination particularly on moving the cervix. Vaginal examination may provoke further bleeding and should probably be delayed until the patient is in hospital if the other features suggest the possibility of a ruptured ectopic.

If implantation occurs in the ampulla there is more room for the pregnancy to expand, and the features are usually those of a leaking ectopic pregnancy:

1. Onset of symptoms usually 6 weeks or more from LMP.
2. Moderate pain in pelvic region usually unilateral, often intermittent.
3. Collapse and serious intraperitoneal blood loss uncommon.

   4. Moderate tenderness and palpable adnexal mass may be present.
   5. Diagnosis may be difficult and is often only made after considerable
   delay.

Management
With a ruptured ectopic, the diagnosis of intraperitoneal haemorrhage is
usually readily made. The patient should be admitted to hospital, using the
obstetric Flying Squad in most cases, and laparotomy should be performed without delay. It is then a simple matter to remove the bleeding
tube. Attempts at resuscitation should not be allowed to delay laparotomy
as the patient is likely to bleed more rapidly than blood can be replaced.

   With a leaking ectopic the diagnosis is more difficult and treatment not
so urgent. An ultrasound scan may establish a diagnosis (or exclude it by
showing a normal intrauterine pregnancy), but in any case of doubt it is
usually better to perform a laparoscopy.

   It is rarely possible or advisable to save the tube involved by the ectopic
pregnancy. Subsequent pregnancies involve at least a 10 per cent risk of
ectopic pregnancy in the other tube. Ectopic pregnancies in sites other
than the tube are so rare that they are of concern only in specialist
practice. Very rarely an ectopic pregnancy implanted elsewhere may
progress and survive to term.

Chapter twelve

Physiology of Pregnancy, Labour and Lactation

Pregnancy produces alterations in the maternal physiology that extend well beyond the obvious changes in the genital tract. All the systems in the body undergo changes, many to produce physiological values totally outside the normal non-pregnant range. While most of these changes can be seen to be directed towards producing a successful fetal outcome, some introduce hazards to the mother, whether or not she starts the pregnancy in normal health. These physiological changes also alter our framework for assessing normal and abnormal organ function. The high steroid output from the ovary and placenta is directly responsible for the majority of the changes, although some of the effects are attributable to the non-steroidal hormones HCG (human chorionic gonadotrophin) HPL (human placental lactogen) and prolactin.

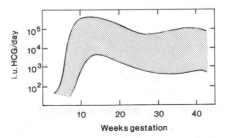

Fig. 12.1. Normal urinary HCG excretion.

Reproductive Hormone Changes

HCG (Fig. 12.1)

HCG is produced by the developing trophoblast and is detectable by sensitive methods from 8 days postovulation, and by routine urine pregnancy testing kits (Pregnosticon, Gravindex) by 35—39 days from the last period (assuming a regular 28-day cycle). Its principal site of action is on the corpus luteum, which is maintained throughout pregnancy and is essential for pregnancy survival until the placenta produces adequate oestrogen and progesterone levels at 7–8 weeks of pregnancy. HCG has an important effect on the male fetus's testicles and less well understood actions on the fetal adrenal gland. In the male fetus it stimulates gonadal production of testosterone (in spite of very high oestrogen influence, which would probably otherwise suppress testicular activity) and this has the effect of producing male differentiation of the genital tract, hypothalamus and cerebral hemispheres.

Progesterone (Fig. 12.2)

Progesterone is the major pregnancy-conserving hormone. It inhibits the release of prostaglandins in the myometrium and decidua and consequently reduces myometrial activity. It also has a generalized smooth muscle

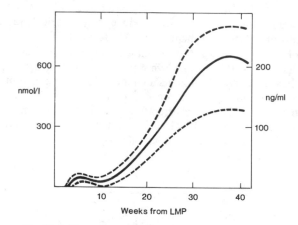

Fig. 12.2. Normal pregnancy, serum progesterone levels.

relaxant effect and numerous metabolic effects, to be outlined below. Until 8–10 weeks progesterone is mainly produced by the corpus luteum (the small peak in the progesterone curve, Fig. 12.2). Thereafter the large majority comes from the placenta. Similar considerations apply to oestrogen production.

Oestrogens (Fig. 12.3)

In pregnancy the placenta produces greatly increased quantities of many oestrogens from fetal and maternal precursors. Oestrone, oestradiol and oestriol, the three main ones, are produced in similar amounts. Oestradiol is the most potent of these and is the major stimulus to growth of the uterus and breasts (although progesterone and other hormones are also important). Oestriol is interesting because it is almost entirely dependent on the fetal adrenal for its precursors. However, its function in pregnancy is unknown, and in rare instances a placental sulphatase deficiency leading

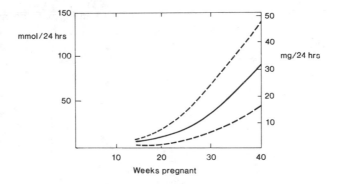

Fig. 12.3. Normal pregnancy, total urinary oestrogen output.

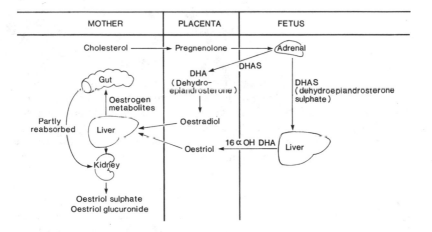

Fig. 12.4. Oestrogen metabolism in the fetoplacental unit.

to an inability to produce oestrogens in the placenta has been found to be compatibile with a normal pregnancy. Maternal metabolism (mainly in the liver and intestine) of the various oestrogens results in a relatively high proportion in both blood and urine being unconjugated oestriol. Oestrogen estimations are widely used in clinical practice as a guide to fetoplacental unit function (*Fig.* 12.4).

HPL (*previously known as HCS – human chorionic somato mammotrophin*) (*Fig.* 12.5)
HPL is produced by the placenta and is detectable from the fifth week of pregnancy. By late pregnancy it is being produced in very large quantities

(up to 3 g/day). It has actions similar to prolactin and growth hormone, is important in the growth and development of the breasts, and may have other functions. It is probably partly responsible for the diabetogenic effect of pregnancy. Serum HPL estimation is also widely used clinically as a placental function test.

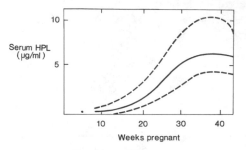

Fig. 12.5. Serum HPL.

Prolactin

Until very recently it was thought that prolactin production was inhibited in pregnancy. It is now known that oestrogen stimulates pituitary production of prolactin, and circulating prolactin levels increase progressively through pregnancy to about 20 times the non-pregnant level by term. Like HPL, prolactin encourages the growth and development of the breasts. Its effect in stimulating lactation is inhibited by the high oestrogen levels of pregnancy.

Relaxin

In pregnancy there is softening of connective tissue and relaxation of ligaments, particularly in the pelvic area. A hormone, relaxin, has been postulated to account for these changes, but it has not been isolated. Some of the effects are certainly due to oestrogen and progesterone and the separate existence of relaxin remains in doubt.

General Endocrine and Metabolic Changes

Thyroid

It is claimed that Egyptian tomb paintings show the use of a tight reed necklace to detect pregnancy thyroid enlargement – possibly the first recorded pregnancy test. Thyroid enlargement in pregnancy is common, particularly in areas with low iodine dietary intake. Otherwise women exhibit many of the features of hyperthyroidism, although remaining essentially euthyroid. The main features of pregnancy thyroid function are:

basal metabolic rate — increased;
protein bound iodine — increased;
thyroxine binding globulin (TBG) — increased;
total T_4 and T_3 — increased;
free thyroxine index — normal;
thyroid-stimulating hormone (TSH) — normal.

The basal metabolic rate increase is due to the high metabolic activity of the fetoplacental unit and the increased maternal cardiac work rate. In common with other binding proteins TBG increases in response to oestrogen, producing higher levels of the bound hormones. Because of this the free thyroxine level is the best index of thyroid function in pregnancy. There is very little passage of thyroid hormones between the fetal and maternal circulations.

Adrenal Function
Corticosteroids
Blood levels and production rates of glucocorticoids increase considerably in pregnancy. Most of the increase in blood levels is in the protein bound portion (due to the increase in corticosterone binding globulin), but free cortisol is also somewhat increased, making the pregnant woman effectively mildly Cushingoid.

Aldosterone
Production and blood levels rise steadily throughout pregnancy to about four times non-pregnancy levels, the increase tending to counteract the sodium losing effect of progesterone.

Carbohydrate Metabolism
Pregnancy may be considered diabetogenic in a number of senses:

1. Some women with previously normal glucose tolerance will become chemical diabetics for the duration of the pregnancy.
2. Normal pregnant women on average produce slightly higher blood sugar levels in a standard glucose tolerance test (and also higher insulin levels).
3. Insulin requirements of diabetic patients generally increase appreciably in pregnancy.

This diabetogenic effect of pregnancy is attributed to HPL, and to the increased steroid output and the increased fat stores of pregnancy, and largely disappears within 48 hours of delivery.

Fasting blood sugar levels are lowered by pregnancy, and the pregnant woman seems to withstand hypoglycaemia better than the non-pregnant.

The renal threshold for glycosuria is commonly lowered in pregnancy due to the large increase in glomerular filtration, and glycosuria hence correlates poorly with blood sugar levels.

Carbohydrate Metabolism in Labour
In labour uterine activity produces increased glucose utilization, and
gastric stasis commonly occurs, leading to a failure of absorption of water
and carbohydrate. In this situation gluconeogenesis occurs with subsequent
production of ketones. Thus ketosis and dehydration are common features
of prolonged labour. They have the important side-effects of impairing
uterine activity, and further prolonging the labour if not corrected, and of
inducing acidosis in the fetus.

Cardiovascular System

Cardiac output increases by an average of about 30 per cent in early
pregnancy with no appreciable change thereafter. (The decrease from 36
weeks that was previously thought to occur is now known to have been an
error produced by the subject's supine position interfering with venous
return.) The increase is explained by proportionate increases in pulse rate
(70 to 85) and stroke volume, and the extra output goes mainly to uterus,
kidneys and skin.

Arterial blood pressure is slightly lowered in normal pregnancy, and
peripheral vascular resistance is substantially lowered — partly by the low
resistance placental vascular bed and partly by a general peripheral vasodilatation — leading to a relatively large fall in diastolic pressure and
an increased pulse pressure. The size of the heart increases radiologically
and the apex beat and the axis of the heart are shifted slightly to the left.
Systolic murmurs are common in pregnancy due to the increased output
and alterations in the walls of the great vessels. Venous engorgement (e.g.
piles and varicose veins) is common, partly because of smooth muscle
relaxation and partly because pressure is high in pelvic and leg veins, due
to uterine obstruction of the inferior vena cava and increased blood flow
from the uterus.

Haematological Changes

The major changes are as follows:

Blood volume increases about 30 per cent.
Plasma volume increases about 45 per cent.
Red cell mass increases about 45 per cent.

Haemoglobin concentration usually falls slightly, although the MCHC
and MCH remain unchanged.

WBC count increases to average $9000/mm^3$ (maximum $16000/mm^3$),
with the increase mainly in neutrophils.

ESR increases to 30–100 mm/hr (but plasma viscosity remains normal).

Iron binding capacity increases, due to the oestrogen-induced increase
in transferrin.

Serum iron concentration falls.

Fibrinogen and factors VII, VIII and X increase substantially, making the pregnant woman's blood hypercoagulable. Fibrinolytic activity decreases.

Respiratory System

The respiratory centre is affected by progesterone from early on in pregnancy and arterial PCO_2 is maintained at about 30 mmHg to 31 mmHg — a level which would result in apnoea in the non-pregnant. In addition the ventilatory response to small increases in PCO_2 is considerably increased, giving rise to the breathlessness of pregnancy. The reduction in PCO_2 is achieved by increased ventilation (+40 per cent) which exceeds the increase in oxygen consumption (+20 per cent). Vital capacity is not affected by pregnancy, but respiration becomes more diaphragmatic than intercostal. The rib cage expands and the diaphragm rises appreciably.

Renal Function and Water Handling

Renal blood flow and glomerular filtration rate increase by 50 per cent in pregnancy. This results in higher clearance rates (normal creatinine clearance in pregnancy 140 ml/min) and diminished blood urea (pregnancy normal 0·4—2·2 nmol/1, 5—13 mg per cent).

The excretion of a water load and the renal handling of sodium are not appreciably altered.

Plasma osmolality is decreased in pregnancy as a result of the diminished PCO_2 and consequent lowering of electrolyte concentration. The resetting of the osmolality centre and subsequent alterations in antidiuretic hormone output may explain the polyuria and polydypsia of early pregnancy.

Water retention occurs in pregnancy over and above that needed for the increase in plasma volume and uterine contents. There is an increase in extracellular fluid, and oedema is common in normal as well as hypertensive pregnancy. It has been amply demonstrated that the presence of oedema in the absence of hypertension is a good sign associated with higher birth weights and decreased perinatal mortality.

There is considerable dilatation of ureters and renal calyces, in pregnancy, due partly to ureteric obstruction and partly to a progesterone relaxant effect. This dilatation, together with increased pregnancy glycosuria leads to an increase in symptomatic urinary tract infection.

Gastrointestinal System

The gastrointestinal tract has not been much studied in pregnancy but there is a widely held belief that it suffers from a progesterone-induced relaxation producing a tendency to heartburn from pyloric and oesophageal reflux, and also gastric stasis in labour, constipation throughout pregnancy and a predisposition to gallstones.

Liver Function

Most standard liver function tests show no change in pregnancy. The exceptions are the serum albumin level, which falls slightly, reducing the albumin/globulin ratio, and the bromsulphthalein test, which may show minimal impairment. However, these tests give a very poor indication of the complex total liver function. It is clear that many aspects of metabolism, depending at least partly on the liver, change radically in pregnancy (e.g. carbohydrate metabolism, clotting function).

Palmar erythema (liver palms) and spider naevi are often found in normal pregnancy and are confined to the parts drained by the superior vena cava. They are presumably related to high oestrogen levels and altered liver function.

Immunological Changes

Modifications in the immune response are necessary to stop the rejection of the placenta by the mother (and vice versa). Cell-mediated immunity is profoundly depressed in pregnancy. This is partly attributable to an oestrogen-induced increase in glycoproteins which coat the lymphocytes with a mucoid layer and partly to the effect of HPL and HCG in suppressing lymphocyte transformation.

Throughout pregnancy fragments of placental tissue (trophoblast emboli) break off into the maternal venous system and probably also play an important part in modifying the maternal immune response.

There is some suggestion that failure of this immune tolerance may produce pre-eclampsia. The depression of immune responses leads to an increased susceptibility to viral diseases and to malaria in pregnancy.

Diagnosis of Pregnancy

Pregnancy may be suspected on the basis of symptoms:

1. delayed menstruation;
2. breast tenderness and fullness;
3. polyuria;
4. tiredness;
5. nausea.

Symptoms (2), (3) and (4) are often (but not always) experienced from the fifth week of pregnancy. Sickness usually appears a week or two later.

Pregnancy may be diagnosed on the basis of physical signs, but before 12 weeks this diagnosis is liable to error except in experienced hands.

The signs are:

1. uterine enlargement (apparent from 6 weeks);
2. uterine softening;
3. increased vascularity — detected by bluish colouring of vagina and cervix, or by arterial pulsation in vaginal fornices;

4. breast changes (pigmentation of the areola and growth of Montgomery's tubercles) — unreliable;
5. Hegar's sign (softening and apparent disappearance to bimanual examination of the uterine isthmus) — unreliable and potentially damaging to elicit.

Diagnostic Tests

The diagnostic tests currently in use depend on the immunological detection of HCG. With clean equipment and modest experience they are highly reliable. They should give a positive result within 25 days of conception (ovulation), but may give negative results after 20 weeks when HCG levels fall. Proprietary kits (Pregnosticon or Gravindex) are suitable for clinic, ward or general practice use.

The Placenta

The process of implantation consists essentially of the invasion of the decidual lining of the uterus by the trophoblast. The decidua is adapted not so much to facilitate this process as to limit it. (Experimentally blastocysts can be made to implant in a large variety of tissues, e.g. eye, kidney or testis, and tend to display tumour-like invasiveness in sites other than the uterus.) In the uterus maternal blood vessels are eroded to form blood-filled spaces (choriodecidual spaces) in which the chorionic villi develop. Septa form more or less distinct compartments into each of which a spiral artery opens, directing blood over a tuft of villi with the blood escaping through veins at the margin of the compartments. Very early in pregnancy the spiral arteries are invaded by trophoblast cells and become appreciably dilated as they approach the placental surface. A high flow, low resistance placental blood supply results so that the chorionic villi are bathed completely in blood with oxygen and carbon dioxide content very close to that of maternal arteries.

The weight of the placenta increases at a different rate to that of the fetus, so that the placenta to fetus weight ratio changes from 4:1 at 10 weeks, to 1:2 at 20 weeks, 1:3·5 at 30 weeks and 1:5 at term.

The placenta has the following functions:

1. production of the hormones, HCG, HPL, oestrogens and progestogens;
2. gas exchange (oxygen and carbon dioxide);
3. nutrition of the fetus;
4. excretion of fetal waste products;
5. anchoring of the fetus;
6. protection of the fetus from immunological attack (cellular immunity and IgM, although the smaller IgG molecules can cross the placenta);
7. heat transfer.

The Fetus

The fetus reaches the size of a jelly baby at 9 weeks, and the size of a (1979!) Mars bar by about 15 weeks. *Crown rump lengths* are shown in *Fig.* 12.6. These can be measured by ultrasound and used for early pregnancy dating to within ± 4 days.

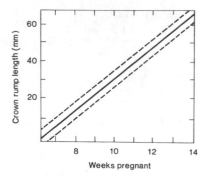

Fig. 12.6. Crown rump lengths in early pregnancy.

The normal range of *biparietal diameters* which are easier to measure and are used for dating later pregnancies is shown in *Fig.* 12.7. It should be noted that the range of normal variation increases from mid-pregnancy and considerably after 28 weeks.

Fetal weight increases (in a sigmoid fashion) throughout pregnancy. It reaches 500 g at about 20 weeks and 1 kg at 28 weeks. Thereafter it increases about 200 g per week to reach 3·3 kg at term (*Fig.* 12.8). The average male fetus weighs about 120 g more than the average female fetus at term.

Organogenesis

The major fetal organs (brain, heart, limbs, kidneys, gut, etc.) develop to something close to their final form between 4 and 9 weeks of pregnancy. Thereafter only minor changes occur in all systems, except the genitalia. Teratogenic substances acting before 4 weeks usually cause death of the embryo; between 4 and 9 weeks they are likely to produce major anatomical defects but after 9 weeks lesser anatomical abnormalities. Functional organ damage may be produced at any stage of pregnancy.

Preparation for Extrauterine Life

Few babies survive with a birth weight below 1000 g or maturity less than 28 weeks, although a baby of 283 g has survived to become a normal child. The mortality rate of babies born alive, but prematurely, in a unit with first-class paediatric care is shown in *Fig.* 12.9 (data from Southmead Hospital, Bristol, 1977–78).

The premature baby may have considerable problems in many different

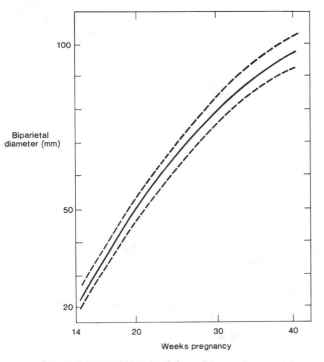

Fig. 12.7. Normal biparietal diameter in pregnancy.

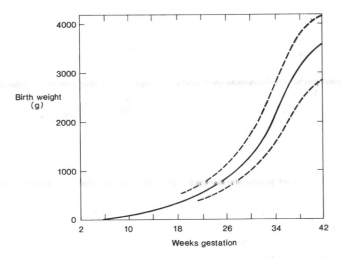

Fig. 12.8. Intrauterine fetal weight. Mean with 10th and 90th percentiles.

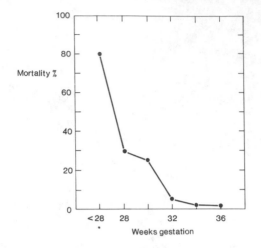

Fig. 12.9. Mortality for all admissions to special care unit, Southmead Hospital, Bristol, 1977—78, related to maturity.

physiological areas (notably breathing, temperature regulation, maintenance of blood sugar, bilirubin handling, combat of infection), but the most common cause of death is functional immaturity of the lungs. The pressure produced by the surface tension of water within the alveoli exceeds the maximum inspiratory effort of the baby and the alveoli cannot expand. To get over this problem, *surfactant,* a substance with detergent properties, is produced in the lungs. Surfactant is usually only produced in significant quantities towards the end of pregnancy, starting anywhere between 24 and 39 weeks.

Corticosteroids can induce surfactant production, and spontaneous labour is usually preceded by several weeks of increased corticosteroid output by the fetus, thus ensuring lung maturity before delivery. It is now possible to measure in amniotic fluid (obtained by amniocentesis) the concentration of lecithin, which is the major component of surfactant. This can give an indication of the functional state of the fetal lung and hence of the likelihood of respiratory distress syndrome (RDS) if the fetus is delivered prematurely. Most laboratories now measure the ratio between lecithin and sphyngomyelin (L/S ratio). Sphyngomyelin production in amniotic fluid is relatively constant during pregnancy so the L/S ratio gives comparable information to the lecithin concentration, and is less influenced by changes in amniotic fluid volume. An L/S ratio of over 2 is associated with a low risk of RDS.

Circulatory Changes at Birth
Within 2 minutes of birth, circulation through the umbilical cord ceases with consequent increase in resistance to outflow from the left side of the

heart. Blood is diverted into the pulmonary circulation, the expansion of the pulmonary vessels being encouraged by respiratory efforts. Both the foramen ovale and the ductus arteriosus close to some extent at this stage, but not totally for several days. This means that it may not be possible to diagnose congenital cardiac anomalies for a few days after birth.

Amniotic Fluid

Amniotic fluid is produced partly by the amnion on the surface of the placenta, but fetal urine output makes a substantial contribution (about 0·5 litre/day at the end of pregnancy). The fetus also swallows appreciable amounts (0·5 litre/day at term) so that disturbances of fetal urine output or of swallowing can produce changes in amniotic fluid volume. There is a net increase in amniotic fluid volume of about 5 ml/day through most of pregnancy. Normal amniotic fluid volume reaches a maximum of about 1—1·5 litres at 36 weeks, diminishing slightly to term and more markedly post term. In the early months of pregnancy the biochemical composition of amniotic fluid closely resembles fetal extracellular fluid, but in the second half of pregnancy it becomes more comparable to fetal urine.

Genital Tract

The size of the uterus and the uterine blood supply increase progressively throughout pregnancy. The weight of the uterus increases from about 60 g (2 oz) in the non-pregnant to 900 g (2 lb) at term.

The uterus entirely fills the pelvis at 14 weeks and from this time tends to rise above the pelvic brim. The position of the fetus is fairly random in the early weeks of pregnancy, constrained only by its tendency to face the placenta. In the middle months of pregnancy the uterus attains an elongated form and the fetus will usually lie with its long axis longitudinally. From about 30 weeks the large majority of fetuses adopt a head down position (cephalic presentation). This is probably because the pelvis acts as a head trap. A fetus presenting as a breech with flexed legs can climb out of the lower uterus, but this may be impossible with a cephalic presentation, or a breech presentation with extended knees (*Fig.* 12.10).

The uterus is divided into upper and lower segments, the lower segment starting at the point where the anterior uterine peritoneum is reflected onto the areolar tissue surrounding the bladder. Functionally the lower segment plays an inactive part in the contractions of labour, being passively stretched upwards and outwards over the presenting part of the fetus. The distinction is of practical importance in Caesarean section operations.

The uterus contracts throughout pregnancy, infrequently early on but with increasing frequency and strength in the weeks preceding the clinical onset of labour. The mother will not usually be aware of these contractions unless she is concentrating. They have the effect of thinning out and expanding (developing) the lower segment of the uterus.

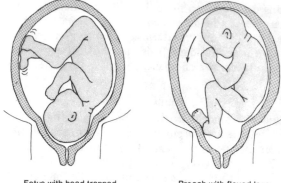

Fetus with head trapped   Breech with flexed legs
and no foothold   able to climb out of pelvis

Fig. 12.10. Head 'trapping' in the last trimester.

Initiation of Labour

The sensitivity of the uterus to oxytocic stimuli alters as term approaches. The factors determining this sensitivity are:

1. The degree of myometrial stretch (increased with twins or poly-hydramnios).
2. The oestrogen/progesterone ratio (increased by oestrogen, decreased by progesterone).

The actual triggering of the onset of labour is brought about by an increase in fetal adrenal activity, probably in response to hypothalamic maturation. This adrenal activity results in increased oestrogen output from the placenta and increased prostaglandin synthesis and release from myometrium and decidua. The increased corticosteroid output also has an important effect in stimulating surfactant production in the fetal lungs. Once labour has started, the strength of contractions is augmented by oxytocin produced by the fetal pituitary and by prostaglandins released in response to cervical stretch and decidual trauma. (There is no significant increase in maternal output of oxytocin in pregnancy or labour.) Dener-vation of the uterus does not stop the normal onset of labour.

First Stage of Labour

Labour is usually assumed to have started when uterine contractions are occurring regularly every 10 minutes or less. The frequency, strength and duration of contractions (and hence the uterine work rate) increase over the first 3 hours or so of labour and then reach a stable state, when contractions will typically occur approximately every 3 minutes, last about a minute and produce an intrauterine pressure around 40 mm Hg. Typical progress of cervical dilatation is shown in *Fig.* 12.11.

In the early stages of labour the cervix becomes effaced or taken up, that is the tubular 'spout' disappears. Thereafter the cervix thins out and dilates progressively (*Fig.* 12.12).

As the cervix and lower segment thin out, the fetal head descends further into the pelvis. This is made easier by moulding of the fetal skull, a process entailing approximation and overlapping of the fetal skull bones, with subsequent diminution of presenting diameters (of more than 1 cm in extreme cases). The maternal pelvis can also 'mould' to some extent,

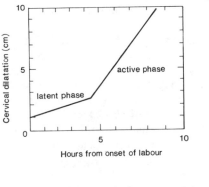

Fig. 12.11. Normal progress of cervical dilatation in labour.

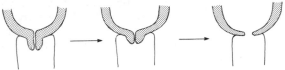

Fig. 12.12. Effacement of the cervix.

thereby increasing pelvic capacity, particularly in the lower pelvis. This is encouraged by the general relaxation of joints and ligaments in pregnancy and is brought about by the woman adopting a squatting or 'pushing' position. Increases in pelvic outlet diameters of over 1 cm are possible.

Second Stage of Labour

When the cervix is fully dilated, descent of the fetal head is more rapid. The mother experiences the urge to bear down (a reflex depending on sensory nerve endings on the pelvic floor and perineum). In the second stage the pelvic floor muscles and fascia surrounding the vagina are progressively dilated by the fetal head. For most women, and primigravidae especially, this entails a lot of hard work.

Contractions usually last over 1 minute at this stage and occur every 2 minutes. Placental blood flow is effectively stopped by contractions in late first stage and second stage and fetal blood oxygen levels and pH tend to fall progressively, making a prolonged second stage undesirable.

Third Stage of Labour

After the delivery of the baby the uterus continues to contract without any appreciable delay. With the first strong contraction the placenta separates from the uterine wall (if it has not already done so during the final expulsion of the baby) by a shearing effect at the level of the decidua spongiosa. The placenta is then gradually expelled from the uterus into the vagina. The placental bed vessels are constricted by the contracted myometrium. Uterine haemostasis is primarily due to this constriction, and the vessels only thrombose as a secondary phenomenon. Clotting disorders will not usually produce excessive uterine blood loss as long as the uterus can contract efficiently and is undamaged.

Uterine contraction in the third stage returns approximately 500 ml of blood from the uterine vasculature into the general circulation, with temporary increase in venous return and central venous pressure. These changes are accentuated by the use of oxytocic drugs, and may be of importance in patients with serious cardiac disease. Ergometrine (but not oxytocin) also produces a rise in blood pressure of 10–20 mm Hg in most patients, with a much larger rise in the occasional patient. For this reason ergometrine is better avoided in patients with serious hypertension.

Lactation

During pregnancy the breasts increase substantially in size (average increase in volume is 250 ml per breast). Oestrogen produces growth of the duct system particularly and progesterone stimulates acinar growth. Prolactin, HPL, insulin, cortisol and thyroxine have also been shown experimentally to be necessary for optimal breast development. Prolactin is the stimulus to lactation and the effect of the high levels of prolactin produced in pregnancy is inhibited until delivery by the high oestrogen levels. Following delivery rapidly falling oestrogen levels allow the onset of lactation. Suckling stimulates further release of prolactin and also stimulates the release of oxytocin which causes contraction of the myoepithelial cells surrounding the alveoli and 'let down' of the milk to the nipple. Basal prolactin levels gradually fall over the course of a few weeks and lactation is maintained by the episodic suckling release of prolactin. Ovarian function is inhibited while high basal levels of prolactin are maintained, but ovulation may resume before lactation ceases so that continued breast-feeding is not a reliable means of contraception.

Further Reading
Hytten F. E. and Leitch I. (1971) *Physiology of Human Pregnancy*. (Introduction by Dugal D. Baird.) Oxford, Blackwell.

Chapter thirteen
Antenatal Care

It has been estimated that at the time of Shakespeare 25 women died out of every 1000 delivered in the City of London. The figure for England and Wales in 1890 was 6·5 per 1000 and in 1973–1975 there were 0·12 deaths directly due to pregnancy and childbirth per 1000 total births (*see* Chapter 16). Perinatal mortality shows the same trend in all developed countries, although their positions in the 'League table' are shifting; at the moment the UK is sliding down the table slightly, possibly due to the restrictions which recurrent financial crises have imposed on the maternity services. Much of this reduced loss of human life is due to generally improving social conditions and to advances in medicine such as blood transfusion and antibiotics. However, there is no doubt that a significant proportion of maternal and perinatal mortality is directly related to the quality of obstetric care. If present trends continue, the obstetric practice of the next generation of general practitioners will, in virtually all cases, be limited to a share of antenatal and postnatal care. There are many complications peculiar to pregnancy; in addition pregnancy affects and is affected by numerous incidental diseases. A sound knowledge of the principles of antenatal care is, therefore, of importance to doctors in most branches of medicine. The fact that such knowledge is not universal, even in the UK, is emphasized by the presence of avoidable factors in 57·8 per cent of the maternal deaths in England and Wales in 1973–1975, many of these representing failure of antenatal care.

The concept of antenatal care has a long and fascinating history, and although Ballantyne is usually credited with its initiation by his publication in 1901 of a 'Plea for pro-maternity hospital', its true origins probably go back much further, in particular to establishments that were primarily concerned with the provision of shelter for the unfortunate women of those days who were illegitimately pregnant. A classic example of such a hospital is the Hôtel Dieu in Paris, and an account of its work was published in 1788. Equal concern for the fetus as for the mother is a very recent development in obstetrics, now that Caesarean section provides a safe alternative for the mother to the difficult and dangerous operative vaginal delivery of former times. Thus even for the specialist obstetrician the relative emphasis placed on antenatal care has increased enormously. Furthermore, the particular concern for the fetus is heightened in labour, when it is at special risk, and continues into the neonatal period. Thus the modern obstetrician needs to be an expert in perinatal medicine.

OBJECTIVES OF ANTENATAL CARE

1. To prevent or detect and treat any abnormalities which threaten the life or wellbeing of the mother or fetus – by regular assessment throughout pregnancy.
2. To prepare her physically for the demands of labour and mother-hood – by advice on diet, exercise and rest, with dietary supplements and drug treatment as necessary.
3. To prepare her psychologically and emotionally for childbearing – developing her confidence in herself and her attendants by personal contact, mothercraft classes and relaxation techniques.
4. To provide opportunities for general health screening – for instance, pregnancy provides an excellent chance to take cervical cytology smears from those most at risk (who are also those least likely to turn up to other cervical smear clinics).

Of these objectives (1), the avoidance of the considerable physical risk of pregnancy, is clearly the most important. It is, however, essential not to lose sight of the other points, and the attainment of all these objectives together should not be impossible.

Place of Delivery

There can be no doubt that the safest place for a woman to be delivered is a fully equipped modern maternity unit. The lower birth rate has meant that this is now possible for virtually all women, whereas 20 years ago patients had to be selected for hospital confinement on the basis of risk factors. General practitioner units attached to major hospitals share these advantages as well as allowing family doctor relationships to flourish. Isolated general practitioner units, however, do not have the facilities to cope with serious emergencies, and their place is now limited to a few geographically isolated areas. When the confinement is normal and the mother and baby fit, early discharge home or to a smaller unit has much to recommend it, combining minimal disturbance of family life with maximum safety. When everything is normal, home confinement can be very satisfying for the family, but it is quite impossible to predict all abnormalities and home confinement entails unnecessary risks to the mother and fetus, even in cases which appear completely normal.

Shared Antenatal Care

Antenatal care can with advantage be shared between the hospital clinic and general practitioner in cases where there are no serious complications (such as diabetes) which would demand constant hospital attendance. With shared care the patient usually has the minimum of travelling while still having access to the expertise and specialized equipment of the hospital, and the general practitioner is able to keep close contact with his patients. Clearly the success of the scheme depends on there being a good working relationship between consultant and general practitioner and on there being adequate communication between the two. This is usually achieved with a personal card (or cooperation card) which the patient herself carries, and on which all important details of the antenatal care are recorded. The patient would normally be seen at hospital for booking early in the pregnancy and then for review on two or three occasions between 28 weeks and term.

Normal Antenatal Care

The normal pattern of antenatal care takes account of the tendency for the major complications of pregnancy (pre-eclampsia, placental failure and antepartum haemorrhage) to occur with increasing frequency as term approaches. Thus the patient is seen monthly until 28 weeks, fortnightly until 36 weeks and then weekly until delivered. Abnormalities in the patient's history or problems developing during the pregnancy may require modification of this scheme.

Booking Clinic

Ideally the patient should attend between 10 and 12 weeks of pregnancy as this is the optimum time for gauging the size of the uterus, and it also allows sufficient time for organizing such measures as insertion of a Shirodkar suture or amniocentesis should these be necessary. A full medical and family history is taken and also a detailed obstetric history. In the medical history heart disease, renal disease, tuberculosis, diabetes, gynaecological operations, drug usage and psychiatric illness are particularly important. Diabetes, tuberculosis and inheritable diseases are of particular consequence in the family history. The obstetric history is of greatest importance because many obstetric problems tend to recur in subsequent pregnancies and may be prevented if anticipated. A general physical examination is carried out, including estimations of weight and blood pressure and urinalysis, and examination of cardiovascular and respiratory systems and the breasts. Abdominal and pelvic examinations are carried out at this visit in order to assess the size of the uterus and to exclude any other abnormal masses. It is particularly important to detect an ovarian cyst if present as this is quite likely to undergo torsion or suffer some other complication during the course of pregnancy (see Chapter 6). A speculum examination is also done and a cervical smear taken, together with appropriate bacteriological swabs should any discharge be present. It is generally inappropriate to attempt to assess pelvic capacity at this stage of pregnancy as it is unpleasant for the patient and also less accurate than an assessment made in late pregnancy when there is a fetal head to act as a 'yardstick'. Pelvic examination properly carried out is not a cause of abortion, but in cases of recurrent abortion it may worry the patient less if the initial pelvic examination is deferred until 13 or 14 weeks.

The following tests are carried out routinely at the booking clinic:

1. Haemoglobin estimation.
2. ABO and rhesus grouping.
3. Antibody screening of rhesus-negative patients.
4. Serological tests for syphilis (VDRL or equivalent).
5. Rubella antibody titres. (80 per cent or more of women will be shown to be immune to rubella and consequently not at risk if exposed to rubella during pregnancy. The remaining patients will need to be investigated further if later exposed to rubella and in any case are usually offered vaccination following the pregnancy.)
6. Haemoglobin electrophoresis to look for haemoglobinopathies in Negroid patients and thalassaemia in those of Mediterranean descent.
7. A midstream urine culture or dip slide for bacteriuria.
8. Cervical cytology smear – if this has not been done within the previous year.

Maturity Assessment

At the first visit a special effort should be made to establish maturity. The expected date of delivery (EDD) is calculated by adding 9 months and 7 days to the date of the first day of the last menstrual period (LMP) e.g. LMP 17.3.79 gives EDD 24.12.79. A note should also be made of:

1. how certain she is of the LMP;
2. whether her cycle is regular;
3. whether she was on oral contraceptives before LMP.

Uterine size is estimated critically to see whether it agrees with maturity calculated from the LMP. If there appears to be any doubt about maturity an ultrasound scan is arranged. It is important that a reliable EDD is arrived at in the first half of pregnancy to enable subsequent growth retardation to be detected (*see* p. 198).

Investigations at Subsequent Visits

1. Haemoglobin estimation. This is usually repeated at least twice during the pregnancy, at about 28 and 34 weeks.
2. Rhesus antibodies are estimated in susceptible patients on two further occasions, usually at 28 and 34 weeks.

Clinical Examination at Subsequent Visits

At each visit it is important to weigh the patient, test the urine for protein and glucose, measure blood pressure, look for signs of oedema and examine the abdomen.

The purpose of the abdominal palpation changes during pregnancy as it becomes possible to detect different features and as different abnormalities become important. The key points looked for are summarized here:

Uterine Size
Throughout pregnancy one is concerned to measure the size of the uterus. If this is greater than expected the following possibilities should be considered:

1. wrong dates;
2. multiple pregnancy;
3. polyhydramnios – excess amniotic fluid (often associated with fetal abnormality);
4. hydatidiform mole (in first half of pregnancy);
5. uterine fibroids;
6. full bladder or rectum in early pregnancy.

If the uterus is small for dates the possible explanations are:

1. wrong dates;
2. placental insufficiency;
3. fetal abnormalities.

The size of the uterus should not simply be gauged by the fundal height. An attempt should also be made to assess the total volume of the uterus, or the actual size of the fetus in late pregnancy.

Fetal Life
Fetal heart sounds may be heard with a stethoscope from about 22 weeks but can be detected with a Doppler ultrasound machine from 10 or 12 weeks of pregnancy. Fetal movements are usually first felt ('quickening') by the primigravid patient between 18 and 22 weeks and by the multigravid patient between 16 and 18 weeks, although there is wide variation.

Fetal Lie
It is not usually possible to detect fetal parts until about 22 weeks, and the fetal lie only becomes clearly definable from about 28 weeks. From 32 weeks the lie should normally be longitudinal and departures from this may merit investigation (*see* p. 193).

Fetal Presentation
The part of the fetus which presents over the pelvis is very variable until 30 weeks, but thereafter it would normally be the head (cephalic presentation), and it becomes important to detect breech presentation from 32 weeks onwards.

Multiple Pregnancy
This may be suspected because of increased size of the uterus from 12 or 16 weeks, but by palpating multiple fetal parts it becomes detectable from about 28 weeks.

Fetal Abnormality

Fetal abnormalities that are not detected by early pregnancy screening may be picked up because of their associated polyhydramnios from 26 or 28 weeks onwards and sometimes because of the small size or abnormal feel of the fetus (for instance, difficulty in feeling a head) from 30 weeks onwards.

Engagement of the Fetal Head

Methods of assessing engagement are described on p. 33 and the implications of non-engagement are discussed on p. 194. It only becomes important in the last weeks of pregnancy.

Position of the Fetal Back

Apart from the detection of the occipitoposterior position, this has no practical value but interests mothers, midwives and occasionally examiners.

Advice in Pregnancy

An important part of antenatal care is the advice given by the doctor and midwife on the subjects below. Booklets are widely available giving common sense advice in terms that most patients will understand, and antenatal classes are organized at most hospital and some community clinics and by organizations such as the National Childbirth Trust. Nevertheless, the doctor should consider it part of his responsibility to talk to the patient on these subjects.

1. Diet

The pregnant woman should eat a well-balanced diet containing plenty of protein (meat, fish, cheese), calcium (milk) and fruit and vegetables to provide vitamins and to combat the tendency to constipation. She does not need to eat large extra quantities of carbohydrate foods. In the UK milk and vitamins are provided at no charge during pregnancy for certain categories of women.

2. Alcohol

Heavy alcohol consumption can produce fetal abnormality or growth retardation. There is no evidence that modest alcohol consumption is harmful.

3. Smoking

Smoking in pregnancy is positively harmful, producing increased perinatal mortality (5 per 1000 excess, in the 1958 Perinatal Mortality Survey), growth retardation and diminished intelligence of surviving children. Strong efforts should be made to persuade the woman to give up smoking completely. As long as she does so in the first half of pregnancy the risk appears to revert to normal.

4. Work
Most women are able to work in their normal jobs during pregnancy until 28 weeks, although complications such as threatened abortion or hypertension may make this inadvisable. Few women work beyond 32 weeks and, unless circumstances are exceptional, patients should be persuaded to give up by this stage.

5. Rest and Exercise
The pregnant woman should not overtire herself at any stage of pregnancy, but can continue to take a moderate amount of exercise throughout. Walking, swimming and cycling can be encouraged, but the more violent forms of exercise should be discouraged, particularly in the later months. Water ski-ing (because of forceful entry of water into the vagina and possibly uterus) can be lethal during pregnancy. In the last trimester an extra few hours of rest in the afternoon is beneficial.

6. Sex
Normal sexual relations may be continued throughout pregnancy unless complications (threatened abortion, antepartum haemorrhage) lead the doctor specifically to advise against it. It is no longer thought necessary to give up 4 weeks before delivery to avoid introducing bacteria into the vagina, but most couples give up at this stage anyway because of the mechanical problems involved.

7. Dental Care
Some degree of gingivitis occurs in about 50 per cent of pregnant women predisposing to caries. For this reason and as a general screening measure every pregnant woman should attend a dentist in pregnancy. Dental care is free during pregnancy and for 12 months afterwards.

8. Financial Benefits
A pregnant woman is entitled to an allowance of £15.70 per week (1979) from 28 weeks for 18 weeks, as long as she has paid full National Insurance contributions in the previous year. Some women also qualify for an earnings related supplement. Some employers offer their own form of additional maternity allowance, or the woman may be able to take maternity leave with full pay if she intends to return to her work following delivery.

In addition, a maternity grant of £25 (1979) per baby is paid to a woman either on her own or her husband's National Insurance contributions in the previous year.

9. Pregnancy, Labour and Delivery
Most women are very interested in what is happening to their bodies during pregnancy, and what will happen to them during labour, what

methods of pain relief are available and so on. A knowledge of these things allows the woman to face her pregnancy with greater confidence. Classes are organized in most centres to impart this type of information and also items (10) and (11).

10. *Mothercraft*
It is helpful for the woman to be taught in advance the rudiments of mothercraft, and also to have sensible guidance about the sort of equipment and clothes she needs to buy for the baby.

11. *Relaxation Techniques*
A number of relaxation techniques are used in the UK and other countries to diminish the pain or discomfort of labour. There can be no doubt that these techniques, if expertly taught, can be of great help to many of those who would have had fairly straightforward deliveries anyway. They cannot, however, overcome all mechanical problems, and there is a danger that some women will have a sense of personal failure to add to the experience of, say, a difficult forceps delivery, if the impression is given that with these methods all women can expect normal painfree deliveries.

Drugs in Pregnancy
The Thalidomide disaster has made the public well aware of the potential for drugs to produce fetal abnormalities. It has also led to the expectation that the medical profession will know which drugs are safe, and to the introduction of legislation allowing legal action to be taken on behalf of a child whose development in utero was impaired by drugs (or other medical action).

In general all drugs should be avoided if possible during the phase of organogenesis (roughly the first trimester, *see* p. 162). Otherwise only drugs known to be safe should be used, and if there is doubt the advice of a pharmacist should be sought. It is not possible to list all drugs problems here but some of the main ones are outlined.

Antiemetics
No adverse reactions are known to the preparations in common use such as Avomine, but a 1980 court decision in the United States accepted the possibility of Debendox being a rare cause of fetal abnormality. Debendox was previously the most wisely used antiemetic in pregnancy.

Antibiotics
Penicillins and cephaloridines are safe throughout pregnancy. Sulphonamides interfere with the bile conjugating mechanism of the neonate and should be avoided if delivery is imminent. Tetracyclines should not be used at all in pregnancy as they stain developing bone and teeth in the fetus and have occasionally produced liver failure in the mother if given

intramuscularly. Streptomycin can cause fetal eighth nerve damage. Trimethoprin is safe after the first trimester (but the sulphonamide warning above applies to the usual sulphonamide–trimethoprin combinations).

Hormones and Related Substances
Progestogens may affect fetal liver function and progestogens of the nortestosterone family (e.g. norethisterone, Primolut N) can cause masculinization of the female fetus. Stilboestrol has been linked to subsequent development of vaginal carcinoma and adenosis in teenagers whose mothers received this drug in pregnancy. Antithyroid drugs in excess can produce cretinism. Corticosteroids generally produce no overt problem, but have been linked with a slight increase in the incidence of cleft palate, and in animals produce some reduction in brain cell division. In very high doses they can initiate labour.

Anticoagulants
Heparin does not cross the placenta and has no fetal effects. Oral anticoagulants do cross the placenta and have been associated with an increased abortion rate in the first trimester, and with fetal cerebral haemorrhage when given within a few days of vaginal delivery.

Sedatives
Barbiturates can be used throughout pregnancy, and are employed to induce fetal liver enzyme production before delivery of those at risk of neonatal jaundice. Phenothiazines, antihistamines and diazepam also appear to be safe, but may cause neonatal depression.

Hypotensives
Methyldopa can be used throughout pregnancy.

Cytotoxic Drugs
Cancer chemotherapy drugs produce embryonic death or malformation when given in early pregnancy and are damaging to the fetus at any stage. Such treatment would usually either be accompanied by therapeutic abortion or delayed until after delivery.

Radiology in Pregnancy
It is now clear that X-ray examination of the pregnant woman involves some risk to the fetus. The work of Dr Alice Stewart in Oxford has demonstrated an excess of leukaemia or other malignant disease in childhood for those irradiated in utero. The magnitude of this risk is of the order of 1 in 30 000 for each abdominal film taken in the second or third trimester and some seven times higher in the first trimester. There is also probably a risk of genetic damage for future generations of comparable order. The recognition of these risks has inhibited the free use of radiology in preg-

nancy. The risks are, however, very small compared with the current perinatal mortality risk (about 18 per 1000, 1978), and if there is a sound clinical indication for an X-ray in pregnancy the benefit is likely to comfortably exceed the risk.

Ultrasound in the dose and frequency range employed diagnostically has not been found to produce any adverse effects in extensive studies, but some degree of caution is necessary until longer term studies have been completed.

ANTENATAL COMPLICATIONS OF PREGNANCY
Abortion

This is dealt with in Chapter 11, but it is worth reminding the reader that patients with a history of middle trimester abortion or of vaginal termination (particularly if past 10 weeks) should be considered for a Shirodkar suture. This is best inserted at around 14 weeks under a general anaesthetic. A single suture of 3 mm nylon tape is inserted in a subserosal plane as high as possible around the substance of the cervix. The patient is usually kept sedated and rested for a few days afterwards to discourage abortion following the procedure (extremely rare). The suture is removed at 38 weeks, or sooner if labour occurs. If this is not done there is a risk of the cervix tearing or of the uterus rupturing in strong labour. It is usually possible to remove the stitch without a general anaesthetic. The Shirodkar suture is a highly successful form of treatment for an incompetent cervix.

Nausea and Vomiting in Pregnancy

Nausea is commonly experienced in early pregnancy, especially between 7 and 12 weeks. It is usually most marked in the morning and abates during the day. Simple dietary measures (such as dry biscuits or toast in bed in the morning, and avoiding fatty foods) allow most women to cope with the nausea without serious vomiting. However, a few patients vomit repeatedly and become ketotic, dehydrated and lose weight. This is called hyperemesis. In previous centuries when there was no effective treatment, such patients would quite probably die from the associated biochemical disturbance or liver failure. (This was the fate of Charlotte Brontë.) Effective treatment is now available, but the incidence of severe vomiting in early pregnancy is also much reduced, underlining the importance of psychological factors in its aetiology.

Patients with vomiting or marked nausea should be treated with anti-emetics. A suitable preparation is Avomine tabs 1 t.d.s. If the vomiting gets worse in spite of these measures the patient should be admitted to hospital for intravenous therapy with saline or glucose saline and correction of any other demonstrable electrolyte imbalance. The nausea and vomiting is always controlled by intravenous therapy. It is a wise psychological move to continue the therapy for at least a day longer than the patient feels is necessary. The patient can usually then be managed satisfactorily with oral antiemetics. Hyperemesis is more common with hydatidiform mole and multiple pregnancy and these should be looked for in every case.

Nausea and vomiting is also sometimes a problem in late pregnancy. It is then often associated with heartburn and reflux oesophagitis. Antacids (mist. mag. trisil. 10 ml as required) will often control both the heartburn and nausea. Sometimes the symptoms are due to reflux of bile salts as a result of pyloric relaxation and they do not respond to any treatment. Vomiting may also be associated with urinary tract infection, and rare incidental causes such as gut or cerebral tumours should be considered in intractable cases.

Fetal Abnormalities

At-risk Cases

Patients at risk of abnormalities are:

1. Those who have had an abnormal child in a previous pregnancy. (This does not include first trimester abortions, virtually all of which are abnormal, as these do not appreciably affect the patient's chances of a subsequent normal term pregnancy.)
2. Patients in their late thirties onwards who are at increased risk of trisomies, particularly Down's syndrome. The risk of producing a mongol is about $1:1000$ at age 25, about $1:100$ at age 38 and $1:50$ at age 45.
3. Those with a family history of inheritable disorders.

Ideally all at-risk patients should have received genetic counselling before the pregnancy and will have a clear idea of the risk of producing a fetal abnormality in this pregnancy, and also of the possibilities of early pregnancy diagnosis of the abnormality concerned. Where appropriate these patients should be offered amniocentesis. Amniocentesis involves the insertion of a fine needle into the uterine cavity under local anaesthetic at about 16 weeks of pregnancy. A preliminary ultrasound makes avoidance of the placenta easier and the whole process safer.

Scope of Amniocentesis

1. Chromosomal abnormalities. After culture of amniotic fluid cells trisomies are detected and also other abnormalities such as Klinefelter's syndrome.
2. Sex-linked conditions (such as haemophilia and Duchenne muscular dystrophy). The sex of the fetus is fairly readily determined, thus revealing the risk of sex-linked conditions (usually no risk for females and $1:2$ for males).
3. Neural tube defects. Liquor alpha feto protein levels give a reliable indication of the presence of open neural tube defects, particularly anencephaly and spina bifida; closed spina bifida will not be detected.

4. Biochemical abnormalities (e.g. Niemann—Pick and Tay—Sachs disease). A number of biochemical abnormalities are detectable by appropriate tests on the cultured cells. The scope of these tests is expanding steadily and up-to-date information must be sought in such cases.

Risks of Amniocentesis

It is possible to damage the placenta, to cause direct damage to the fetus or possibly to provoke an abortion. Such risks are largely avoided by the prior use of ultrasound. The overall risk of damaging a normal fetus or of producing an abortion is probably of the order of 1 : 200 in experienced hands. Amniocentesis is usually offered to women when the chance of finding an abnormal fetus is at least 1 : 100. This includes all those over 38 years.

Fetoscopy

It is possible to insert a small endoscope through the abdominal wall and through the uterine wall into the amniotic cavity to directly visualize the fetus in early pregnancy, and to obtain fetal blood from the placental surface. It is not yet certain that the risks of this procedure do not outweigh its advantages, and as the indications are few it should only be performed in very few hospitals where experience will be concentrated.

Ultrasound

Expert ultrasound examination can detect spinal abnormalities (even closed lesions) in the first half of pregnancy and various other abnormalities at later stages, but the necessary equipment and expertise is not yet generally available.

Routine Screening of Normal Patients

Routine screening of all antenatal patients by maternal serum alpha feto protein levels has been introduced in a number of units. The blood test needs to be done between 16 and 20 weeks. The top 3 per cent of the population range includes the majority of the open neural tube defects, a much larger number of normal pregnancies, most of the twin pregnancies and a substantial number of cases where the estimated maturity is wrong. Consequently only 1 : 20 of those with abnormal serum alpha feto protein levels will have an abnormal fetus. An abnormal serum alpha feto protein indicates the need for an ultrasound examination to confirm maturity and exclude twins and to identify placental site, and this may be followed by an amniocentesis where appropriate. Because of the involvement of large numbers of normal pregnancies, a normal fetus is likely to be aborted occasionally by mistake, so the overall benefits of the procedure are not as clear cut as might be hoped.

Fetal Abnormalities in Later Pregnancy
A fetal abnormality should be suspected in the following situations:

1. polyhydramnios;
2. where the uterus is small for dates;
3. when the fetus feels abnormal, particularly if there is difficulty feeling a head.

If there is serious suspicion of fetal abnormality an ultrasound examination or a straight abdominal X-ray should be done. Biochemical tests are not generally helpful in establishing fetal abnormality in late pregnancy.

Where major fetal abnormalities are detected the obstetrician will normally elect to induce labour; if it is appreciably before term, prostaglandin infusion is the method of choice (*see* Chapter 8). Fetal abnormalities may present mechanical difficulties in labour, the most common problem being disproportion with a hydrocephalic fetus. In such instances the enlarged fetal head may have to be decompressed by introducing a catheter through the associated spina bifida with a breech presentation or by directly draining the head with a wide bore needle. Fetuses with significant hydrocephalus always have grossly damaged brains and should not be considered salvageable.

Genetic Counselling
Patients who have just had an abnormal fetus or who are at risk for other reasons should be offered counselling by specialist genetic counsellors who are available in most areas. Where such a service is not available an interested obstetrician can give appropriate advice. The essential basis for genetic counselling is an accurate diagnosis of the type of abnormality that has already occurred; therefore all abnormal fetuses should be subjected to post-mortem examination. The principles of deriving risk estimates for most conditions are simply explained in *Genetic Counselling* by Stevenson and Davison (1978).

For the most common major CNS abnormalities (anencephaly, spina bifida and hydrocephalus) the risk of recurrence is about 1:30, rising to 1:10 if two previous children have been affected.

Multiple Pregnancy
In the UK the incidence of twins is about 1:80, the incidence of triplets about $1:80^2$, of quadruplets $1:80^3$ and so on. The practice of induction of ovulation with clomiphene and gonadotrophins produces an increased chance of multiple pregnancy, particularly of the high multiple pregnancies in association with gonadotrophin induction (*see* Chapter 11). The incidence of multiple pregnancy varies in other populations, being higher, for instance, in Nigerians and lower in the Chinese.

Twins may develop from the same ovum (then called uniovular, monozygotic or identical) or from two ova fertilized at the same time (binovular, dyzgotic or non-identical). If they derive from the same ovum there is a possibility that they share the same placenta, chorion and amnion depending on the stage at which division occurs. Those sharing the same amnion are floating in the same amniotic sac and stand a great risk of cord entanglement. This situation is fortunately very rare, but it is relatively common to find identical twins sharing the same chorion. Non-identical twins never share the amnion, chorion or placenta although fusion of two separate placentae is common. Examination of the placenta and membranes only gives a certain guide to the zygosity of twins of the same sex when the membranes are monochorionic (*see Fig.* 13.1).

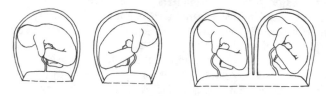

Dichorionic
Diamniotic

Can be either. About ⅙ same sex twins are identical

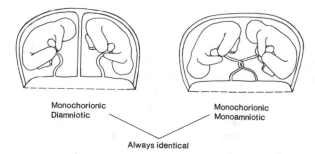

Monochorionic   Monochorionic
Diamniotic   Monoamniotic

Always identical

Fig. 13.1. Placental arrangement in twin pregnancy.

Some mixing of the placental circulation is also common with identical twins sharing the same placenta and this will occasionally lead to unequal blood flow with one infant becoming plethoric and the other grossly anaemic and undernourished, sometimes dying in utero. There is also the risk of exsanguination of the second twin during delivery if the cord of the first twin is allowed to bleed.

Higher multiple pregnancies are usually derived from multiple ovulation, but sometimes one or more of the siblings are identical.

Diagnosis
There should be increased suspicion of multiple pregnancy when there is a family history of twins, a history of induced ovulation, or of hyperemesis,

although usually none of these factors is present. Clinical signs are more helpful, and the most important of these is the finding of increased uterine size or growth rate. The palpation of multiple fetal parts is also a fairly reliable sign later in pregnancy. However, multiple pregnancy can rarely be diagnosed with certainty on the basis of clinical signs alone and whenever it is suspected an ultrasound scan should be arranged. After 32 weeks an ultrasound diagnosis of multiple pregnancy should be confirmed by X-ray, as triplets are often misdiagnosed as twins by ultrasound.

Complications of Multiple Pregnancy
Almost every complication of pregnancy is more common with twins and the risks increase with higher numbers of fetuses. Prematurity is so common that multiple pregnancy accounts for 15 per cent of all premature deliveries. Placental insufficiency is another serious hazard; twins tend to be small for dates and triplets more so. The 1958 Perinatal Mortality Survey showed that 3·5 per cent of all twins died of intrauterine asphyxia (mostly associated with placental failure). Because of greater requirements deficiencies of iron, calcium and folic acid are common unless supplements are given. Acute pyelonephritis, pre-eclampsia, polyhydramnios and malpresentation are also more common. The greater placental area means that placenta praevia is more likely. The minor problems of pregnancy such as backache, piles, varicose veins and dyspepsia are more common and troublesome.

Management
The most important part of management is the early diagnosis of multiple pregnancy. Iron and folic acid supplements should be given and frequent checks made on haemoglobin levels. The patient should be advised to make special efforts to get adequate rest and will normally be seen more frequently at the antenatal clinic. Some units routinely admit such patients between 28 and 32 weeks for hospital bed rest in the hope of reducing the incidence of prematurity, but there is no evidence that this is effective. Early admission in cases of suspected premature labour may allow prolongation of the pregnancy (*see* p. 196). Minor departures from normality (particularly in blood pressure) will be treated seriously and usually result in hospital admission. Many obstetricians feel that twins should not be allowed to go past 38 weeks because of the danger of placental insufficiency and all are agreed that they should not go past term. The patient should, of course, be booked for delivery in a specialist obstetric unit because of the increased likelihood of intrapartum difficulties (see Chapter 14).

Breech Presentation
Breech presentation is abnormal after 32 weeks. About 25 per cent of fetuses present by the breech at 30 weeks but most undergo spontaneous version leaving only about 3 per cent as breech presentations by 36 weeks.

The main aetiological factors in persistent breech presentation are as follows:

1. fetal legs extended at the knees;
2. multiple pregnancy;
3. uterine abnormalities;
4. fetal abnormalities, particularly hydrocephalus and spina bifida;
5. polyhydramnios;
6. oligohydramnios.

The terms used to describe the various positions of the fetal legs are illustrated in *Fig.* 13.2. The extended breech is especially common in the primigravida and is associated with a somewhat longer first and second stage of labour. The flexed breech is associated with a shorter labour but a higher incidence of cord prolapse. The overall risk to the fetus is not

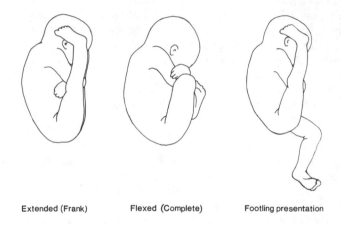

Extended (Frank)   Flexed (Complete)   Footling presentation

Fig. 13.2. Terms used to describe the position of the legs in breech presentation.

appreciably different with either type of breech and there is no justification for treating one form of breech differently from the other. (In the past some obstetricians have been more inclined to do elective Caesarean sections for flexed breeches.) The fetus presenting by the breech is at increased risk for two main reasons:

1. The fetal head does not pass through the pelvis until the body has been delivered so that no time is allowed for moulding and there is no opportunity to opt for Caesarean section if the head proves to be too big to go safely through the pelvis.
2. Intrauterine asphyxia is more common because of cord problems (partly cord prolapse but also cord compression and entanglement as the thighs are compressed against the abdomen in the first stage of

labour), and partly due to cord compression and impairment of placental blood flow in the minutes between the delivery of the umbilicus and the delivery of the head.

Because of the lack of time for moulding to occur an appreciably larger pelvis is needed to deliver a baby safely as a breech than as a vertex. A good shaped pelvis with an obstetric conjugate of over 11·5 cm is needed to deliver safely the average sized term baby.

With modern management methods the perinatal mortality for vaginal breech delivery should not exceed 1 per cent (for mature normal babies).

Management of Breech Presentation

After 32 weeks it is essential positively to identify the head at each examination. If this is not possible on abdominal examination, a vaginal examination should be made to feel for a deeply engaged head, and if the head is still not found an ultrasound scan or an X-ray is indicated, as breech presentation or anencephaly are likely in such circumstances. Consideration should be given to attempting external cephalic version on breech presentations at 34 weeks. The risks of external version are:

1. bruising of the uterus or premature rupture of membranes leading to premature labour;
2. traumatic detachment of the placenta (abruption);
3. cord entanglement leading to fetal distress;
4. fetomaternal bleeding leading to sensitization of rhesus-negative mothers.

External version is contraindicated in:

1. the hypertensive patient (risk of abruption);
2. any antepartum haemorrhage;
3. multiple pregnancy;
4. previous Caesarean section;
5. any situation where the patient is destined to have a Caesarean section in any case.

Provided that case selection is good and no undue force is used, and the patient is not anaesthetized, the overall risk of external version is minimal. However, if the risk of breech delivery continues to lessen, it is likely that the risks of version will exceed the difference between that of breech and vertex delivery and hence version will become unjustifiable. If fetal distress occurs after external version (and one should always listen to the fetal heart following version) then the fetus should be turned back to its original position.

When a breech presentation persists after 36 weeks and where reasons for Caesarean section do not already exist, a pelvic assessment should be made. This is done partly by vaginal examination and partly by lateral

X-ray pelvimetry. It is also a help to assess the size of the fetal head by ultrasound cephalometry. If these procedures show that there is ample room for the fetus then a vaginal breech delivery should be aimed for; otherwise an elective Caesarean section should be planned.

Some obstetricians advocate induction of labour at 38 weeks for breech presentation to limit the size of the baby, but the place of this is debatable. Breech delivery is described in Chapter 14.

Malpresentations Other than Breech

Brow and face presentations are rarely diagnosed in the antenatal period and are dealt with in Chapter 14.

Pre-eclampsia and Eclampsia

Pre-eclampsia was traditionally defined as a disease process occurring in pregnancy where two out of the three cardinal signs of hypertension, proteinuria and oedema are found. This is not a satisfactory definition, and a better one would be a disease process arising usually in the second half of pregnancy, characterized by hypertension and in all except mild cases by proteinuria and usually, but not always, by oedema. There is still some uncertainty about the aetiology of pre-eclampsia although recent work has thrown much interesting light on this. There can be no doubt that most of the pathology of pre-eclampsia is due to intravascular coagulation, and there is some suggestion that failure of immune tolerance between the mother and fetus may play some part in its aetiology (see Further Reading). Pre-eclampsia is more common —

in primigravidae;
in multiple pregnancy;
in cases of essential hypertension;
in diabetes;
in cases of hydatidiform mole.

This last condition is the only situation in which pre-eclampsia occurs in the first half of pregnancy.

The course of pre-eclampsia varies appreciably from case to case. Some patients maintain a mild elevation of blood pressure over a number of weeks without developing albuminuria, whereas others rapidly develop albuminuria and worsening hypertension and go on to eclampsia if not treated promptly. In general, the earlier the onset of pre-eclampsia in the pregnancy the more serious is the outlook. Albuminuric pre-eclampsia produces serious impairment of placental function leading to growth retardation or intrauterine death, and a five to sixfold increase in perinatal mortality. Non-albuminuric pre-eclampsia only marginally increases the risk to the fetus.

Eclampsia is the occurrence of fits in a pre-eclamptic patient. It is virtually confined to albuminuric cases. The tendency to fit is not clearly related to the degree of hypertension and is probably caused by local cerebral anoxia produced by plugging of small cerebral vessels with fibrin. Eclampsia and severe pre-eclampsia are often associated with:

1. impaired liver function sometimes with subcapsular haemorrhage;
2. impaired renal function often with oliguria and sometimes anuria;
3. intravascular coagulation, occasionally sufficient to cause coagulation disorders;
4. impaired lung function;
5. generalized oedema, including glottal oedema sometimes leading to difficulty in anaesthetizing such patients.

Eclampsia due to untreated pre-eclampsia was probably the major cause of maternal mortality in the past, but it should now be considered a preventable disease. However, a considerable proportion of perinatal mortality is still attributable to pre-eclampsia. Diagnosis is usually easy as long as the patient is seen regularly and blood pressure recording and urinalysis are carried out at each visit. Most failures of modern management occur because of failure to act at the first sign of pre-eclampsia rather than failure to elicit these signs.

Management
There is no cure for pre-eclampsia apart from termination of the pregnancy (with the attendant risk to the fetus of premature delivery). The essential part of management of the condition is close observation of the patient to determine whether intervention is necessary in the interests of mother or fetus, or whether the pregnancy can be allowed to proceed. It is usual to admit patients with pre-eclampsia to hospital for this observation. Safe management of pre-eclampsia at home is not really possible. There is some evidence that bed rest improves placental function and hence adds to the fetal safety, but this is not the primary object of hospital admission. Observation includes frequent blood pressure measurements, estimation of proteinuria, placental function tests (*see* p. 199), and in moderate or severe pre-eclampsia estimation of renal function, particularly by serum uric acid levels. If there is serious deterioration of the condition of the mother or the fetus she must be delivered. Hypotensive agents, diuretics and sedatives have no effect on the underlying disease process and indeed may increase the risk to the fetus by reducing placental perfusion. Thus they have little place in the long-term management of pre-eclampsia. They do, however, have an important role in the short-term emergency treatment of eclampsia or severe pre-eclampsia.

Emergency Treatment of Eclampsia or Severe Pre-eclampsia
The emergency treatment of eclampsia is similar to that of severe pre-eclampsia once the decision to terminate the pregnancy has been taken. It

is essential in the first instance to control the fits or fitting tendency. This is effectively done by intravenous injection of diazepam 10 to 20 mg followed by slow intravenous infusion of diazepam (Valium) 40 mg in 1 litre of glucose saline. To control the blood pressure, hydrallazine 40 mg per litre may be added to the same infusion bottle. It has been traditional to nurse the eclamptic patient in a darkened, quiet room but the diazepam—hydrallazine regime makes normal labour ward conditions acceptable. Once established on this regime the patient would normally be delivered without further delay. If the situation is particularly favourable for vaginal delivery this might be achieved by induction of labour, but in most instances the delivery method of choice would be Caesarean section. A close watch is kept on urinary output. If this falls, intravenous frusemide or mannitol may be needed. If the woman is allowed to labour, very close observation of her condition and that of the fetus is necessary. She should not be allowed to push in the second stage of labour, the baby being delivered electively by forceps or ventouse. Ergometrine should be avoided following delivery because of its tendency to induce hypertension. Syntocinon 5 units i.m. is a safe alternative. The eclamptic regime should be continued for 24 hours following delivery and a reduced level of sedation should then be used for several further days. Following delivery of the placenta the patient's condition tends to improve with a diminution of blood pressure and a tendency to diuresis. The blood pressure may not, however, return entirely to normal for several weeks or even months following delivery.

Treatment of Eclampsia Occurring at Home
If possible the patient should be restrained during the fit so that she does not hurt herself by hitting hard objects. She should be turned on to her side and her airway checked. The fit should be stopped with an injection of diazepam 10 to 20 mg i.v. if this is available (i.m. if an intravenous injection is not possible). Other anticonvulsants can be used if diazepam is not available. The obstetric flying squad should be called to the patient's home. This is safer for her than sending her into hospital. She should not be left unattended while waiting for the flying squad.

Prognosis for Future Pregnancies
The patient with pre-eclampsia in her first pregnancy has approximately a 1 : 3 chance of having pre-eclampsia in her next pregnancy. It is probable, however, that the pre-eclampsia will be less severe and later in onset. This means that the outlook for subsequent pregnancies is generally quite good even when the woman has lost her first baby because of pre-eclampsia arising very early in pregnancy. Virtually all women with recurrent pre-eclampsia are destined to become chronic hypertensives.

Antepartum Haemorrhage

This is defined as bleeding from the genital tract from 28 weeks of pregnancy until delivery. Bleeding before 28 weeks is classed as a threatened abortion, although the causes and treatment of bleeding between week 20 and week 28 are broadly similar to those of antepartum haemorrhage (APH). Antepartum haemorrhage may be due to:

1. placenta praevia;
2. placental abruption or accidental haemorrhage (premature separation of a normally situated placenta);
3. bleeding from other parts of the genital tract;
4. vasa praevia.

Clinical Features

1. *Placenta Praevia*

Bleeding from a placenta praevia is typically painless, recurrent and usually unprovoked (although it may occasionally follow intercourse). The amount lost may vary between a few spots and several pints. If the patient is shocked the degree of shock is proportional to the visible blood loss. The uterus is usually well relaxed and the fetal parts readily palpable, with the presenting part usually not engaged and sometimes deviated to one side. Except in the most severe cases, where there is marked maternal shock, the fetal heart is present.

2. *Placental Abruption*

In abruption the bleeding may be partly or totally concealed as blood accumulates in the fundus of the uterus before tracking down to the cervix. In minor cases there may be no features to distinguish the bleeding from that of a placenta praevia, but in moderate or severe cases there is typically pain with or preceding the bleeding. In some instances the patient presents with severe pain and shock before there is any visible bleeding, and the patient may be shocked out of proportion to the external blood loss. Typically the uterus is tense and tender and it may be impossible to feel fetal parts. In all except minor cases the fetal heart is often already absent when the patient is seen. When the patient is examined under anaesthesia it is often found that the fetal head is deep in the pelvis, and the cervix is appreciably dilated. In the more severe cases a consumption coagulopathy may develop with hypofibrinaemia and sometimes also excessive fibrinolysis. Placental abruption may be caused by trauma (e.g. road accidents or external version) and is more common with severe hypertensives but in most cases there is no clear aetiology. Folic acid deficiency has been suggested as a cause but the evidence is unconvincing.

3. *Other Genital Tract Bleeding*

Antepartum haemorrhage may also arise from a cervical polyp, a cervical carcinoma, a circumvallate placenta or trauma (possibly self-induced). A cervical 'erosion' may also occasionally bleed slightly following intercourse or instrumentation. A careful speculum examination should reveal most of these sources of bleeding, but it is not safe to assume that a polyp or erosion is a source of bleeding until the more serious possible sources have been excluded.

4. *Vasa Praevia*
Very rarely bleeding may occur from an abnormal fetal vessel attached to the membranes over the internal os in velementous insertion of the cord. Such bleeding virtually only occurs following artificial rupture of the membranes or during labour.

Management of Antepartum Haemorrhage
Unless there is clear clinical evidence of placental abruption the bleeding should be assumed to be coming from a placenta praevia until proved otherwise. There is no place for vaginal examination until the fetus is sufficiently mature and circumstances are suitable for immediate delivery by Caesarean section should such an examination reveal a placenta praevia, as it may provoke heavy bleeding. All cases of antepartum haemorrhage should be transferred at once to a major obstetrical unit. Unless the bleeding is minimal the flying squad should be called. Once in hospital it is usual to carry out a gentle speculum examination to visualize (but not touch) the cervix to see whether the blood is coming through the os (that is to say from the placenta) or whether it arises from a source in the cervix or vagina. One should not wait until the bleeding has ceased, because even if a cervical lesion is found one cannot then be certain that it was the actual source of bleeding. Provided that the bleeding is not heavy and settles down within a day or two it is usual to attempt to locate the placenta (nowadays usually by ultrasound but previously by soft-tissue radiography, arteriography or isotope scanning). Placental function tests are also carried out. If the placenta can be reliably shown to be normally situated and placental function is unimpaired the patient may be allowed home (although this is one of the few instances when it is certainly wise to advise against coitus for the rest of the pregnancy). If placenta praevia cannot be excluded, the initial bleed was a substantial one, or the bleeding recurs, the patient should remain in hospital until delivered. In the case of repeated or heavy bleeding it may be necessary to deliver the fetus by Caesarean section immediately, but otherwise it is normal to aim to deliver the patient at 38 weeks (appropriate steps having been taken to confirm fetal maturity). At 38 weeks the patient is examined under anaesthesia to confirm or exclude the presence of a placenta praevia. This is done in theatre with blood cross-matched and staff and instruments ready to carry out immediate Caesarean section, in case vaginal examination should provoke heavy bleeding. If a placenta praevia is confirmed the treatment is immediate Caesarean section. It should be noted that in the presence of

a placenta praevia this may be an extremely vascular, difficult and hazardous operation and should only be undertaken by experienced obstetric staff. If a placenta praevia is not found at the time of examination under anaesthesia it is probably best to induce labour by rupturing the membranes, as there is a possibility that the bleeding will have damaged placental function or may recur more severely if the patient is left to labour spontaneously.

In conclusion it should be re-emphasized that the complaint of antepartum haemorrhage must be taken very seriously and the patient transferred at once, and by flying squad if necessary, for proper investigation and treatment without any pelvic examination having been carried out at home. There is no place for waiting to see whether it happens again. Disaster may be only a blood clot away.

Management of Placental Abruption

Minor degrees of placental abruption cannot usually be diagnosed and their management is as outlined above for antepartum haemorrhage in general. However, major degrees of abruption are usually readily diagnosed and have their own form of management. The flying squad should be called and the patient transferred to a major obstetric unit – unless, of course, she is already there.

An intravenous infusion should be started and at least 4 units of blood cross-matched. A central venous pressure line is invaluable in managing severe abruption, and without one most such patients will be undertransfused. When the patient is first seen, blood should be taken for clotting function tests, particularly fibrinogen concentration. This can be done formally in the laboratory if a suitable service is available, but information which is almost as valuable can be gained from observing clot formation in a plain glass tube at the bedside. If a firm clot has not formed within 10 minutes of taking blood it is reasonable to assume that the patient has hypofibrinogenaemia. If a clot forms and subsequently becomes friable it is likely that she has excessive fibrinolytic activity. Such clotting function tests should be repeated at intervals until after the patient has been delivered.

The patient is best transfused with fresh blood (if it is available) in order to replenish depleted clotting factors. It is probably unnecessary to treat hypofibrinogenaemia or excessive fibrinolysis specifically unless the patient is actively bleeding, but if there is appreciable active loss then fibrinogen may be replaced with a pure fibrinogen solution or with fresh frozen plasma. Excessive fibrinolysis may be treated with epsilon – aminocaproic acid (Epsikapron).

Once the patient's condition has been assessed and a transfusion has been started, labour is induced by rupturing the membranes and starting a syntocinon infusion if necessary. Rupturing the membranes allows a more ready drainage of blood from the uterine cavity and discourages further tracking of blood into the myometrium with release of thromboplastic substances into the circulation. Most patients with severe abruption labour readily and deliver without undue delay. If the fetus is alive it should be monitored closely. There is a very serious risk of postpartum haemorrhage in these cases and many of the deaths associated with placental abruption are attributable to postpartum haemorrhage occurring in patients already hypovolaemic from antepartum haemorrhage. The uterus may be badly bruised by blood tracking out from the retroplacental space into the myometrium, and this bruising interferes with uterine contraction in the third stage of labour. If, in addition, there is clotting dysfunction, then the scene is set for a brisk postpartum haemorrhage which is difficult to control and may readily prove fatal. In such circumstances the delivery must not be left to inexperienced junior staff. Intravenous ergometrine will be given and syntocinon added to the drip. Haemorrhage may have to be controlled by bimanual compression of the uterus and any clotting abnormality should be corrected at this stage.

Acute renal failure and pituitary necrosis leading to Sheehan's syndrome are both possible complications of severe placental abruption, but careful attention to blood volume replacement aided by central venous measurement should avoid these complications.

Polyhydramnios

Polyhydramnios (often abbreviated to hydramnios) is the presence of excess amniotic fluid in the uterine cavity. Volumes of amniotic fluid up to 1·5 litres are normal in the last trimester. However, it is not easy to measure amniotic fluid volume, so the diagnosis of polyhydramnios is a clinical one based on the following features:

1. a uterus which is large for dates and tense;
2. difficulty in palpating fetal parts;
3. a fluid thrill;
4. unstable lie.

Acute and chronic forms of hydramnios are described. The relatively rare *acute polyhydramnios* is typically associated with fetal abnormality or uniovular twins. There is often a rapid onset of uterine distension in the late second trimester or early third trimester with abdominal discomfort, and a high incidence of premature labour. The patient is best admitted to hospital, and an X-ray should be taken to exclude bony fetal abnormality. If the fetus appears normal, steps should be taken to prevent premature labour (*see* p. 196) but are likely to be unsuccessful.

The more common *chronic polyhydramnios* is associated with fetal abnormality (particularly gut atresia or anencephaly), maternal diabetes and multiple pregnancy, but often no cause is found. It generally presents slightly later in pregnancy and is not very commonly associated with maternal discomfort or premature labour. Abdominal X-ray and a glucose tolerance test will generally be performed. However, with the lesser degrees of hydramnios the patient need not be admitted to hospital until the onset of labour, but she should be warned to come into hospital early on in labour or immediately the membranes rupture. Polyhydramnios presents the following dangers in late pregnancy and labour:

1. possible unstable lie with malpresentation;
2. rupture of membranes with cord prolapse;
3. placental abruption due to the sudden reduction in uterine size following drainage of large volumes of liquor.

A close watch should be kept on the presentation in such cases and the patient should be warned to come into hospital early in labour. If the membranes are ruptured artificially this should be done in a controlled fashion to release the liquor slowly over the course of several minutes. Control can be achieved partly by pressing down the fetal head into the brim and partly by obstructing the vagina with the examining fingers. When an apparently normal baby is delivered to a woman with poly-hydramnios a stomach tube should be passed without delay to exclude the possibility of oesophageal atresia as there is a serious danger that the baby will drown in its first feed, if the oesophageal atresia is not detected.

Oligohydramnios

Oligohydramnios is associated with failing placental function, with post-maturity and with the rare cases of fetal genitourinary abnormalities preventing urine output (particularly renal agenesis). The diagnosis is suggested by the clinical impression that the uterine wall is wrapped closely around the baby with no intervening liquor. This finding should lead one to assume that the placenta is failing and to institute urgent investigations (*see* p. 199).

Unstable Lie (Variable Lie)

It is normal for the fetal lie to be longitudinal from 32 weeks onwards. An unstable (or variable) lie is only of clinical importance in the last few weeks of pregnancy. The causes are:

1. high parity, with associated lax uterine and abdominal muscles;
2. hydramnios;
3. uterine abnormalities;
4. rarely, pelvic 'tumours' such as placenta praevia, cervical fibroids or an ovarian cyst incarcerated in the pelvis.

With an unstable lie there is a danger that labour will start, or that the membranes will rupture while the fetus is lying transversely, which may lead to cord prolapse with the possibility of fetal death, or to the prolapse of an arm which fixes the fetus in an undeliverable position. It is advisable to admit the patient with an unstable lie from 38 weeks onwards to hospital to await the onset of labour. At the first sign of labour the patient is examined and, if possible, the presentation corrected to cephalic. Should the membranes rupture while the lie is unstable a vaginal examination should be performed to exclude cord prolapse.

Abnormal Lie

Some patients will be found to have a persistently abnormal lie in which the fetus lies in the same abnormal position without change. The causes of this are rather different from those of the truly unstable lie. Pelvic 'tumours' and more marked degrees of uterine abnormality are the more likely causes. The management is broadly similar to that of other forms of unstable lie, but should it prove impossible to correct the lie at the onset of labour then a Caesarean section will be necessary. Caesarean section for a transverse lie may have to be done through a classical incision rather than a lower segment incision but should only be undertaken by an experienced operator.

Disproportion

Disproportion exists when some part of the fetus is too big to pass through the maternal pelvis. The fetal head is usually the largest part of the fetus in cross-section, and disproportion usually refers to cephalopelvic disproportion. In a few instances, however, the shoulders may be larger than the fetal head, and shoulder dystocia (which is difficulty in delivering the shoulders after the head has delivered) is a special form of disproportion.

Disproportion was a common and very serious obstetric problem in previous centuries, accounting for much maternal mortality and morbidity. With women living in poverty, rickets was common; this frequently caused gross distortion and contraction of the pelvic inlet with obstetric conjugates sometimes as little as 5 cm, making delivery of any sized baby impossible. In such circumstances the woman would be likely to die a biochemical death after some days in labour, or alternatively might rupture her uterus and die more swiftly from blood loss. Those with lesser degrees of pelvic contraction might eventually manage to deliver a dead and partly collapsed fetus and then suffer total urinary or faecal incontinence because of pressure necrosis of the vaginal wall and bladder or rectum. Before the introduction of Caesarean section as a moderately safe procedure at the end of the last century a wide range of gruesome instruments were used to destroy the fetus and deliver it piecemeal in order to save the mother. Even in the most skilled hands the mortality and morbidity of these destructive operations was still high.

The virtual disappearance of malnutrition has meant that disproportion is uncommon and it now occurs in less than 1 per cent of deliveries. Nowadays disproportion is only likely in cases where the pelvis is distorted due to bony disease such as lumbar kyphoscoliosis or a displaced fracture of the pelvic brim or outlet especially from a road traffic accident, or alternatively where the fetus is unduly large (as with poorly controlled diabetes or hydrocephalus). In the absence of such abnormalities disproportion is rare in women over 5 ft 1 in (154 cm) and it is very rare in women who have previously had normal vaginal deliveries (although not totally unknown). In the past much time and effort has been spent trying to predict disproportion in primigravidae by both clinical and radiological methods. However, the variable degree of moulding of the fetal skull and maternal pelvis, the variable resistance of the maternal soft parts and the variable efficiency of uterine action make prediction of disproportion unreliable except in gross cases. There is a growing tendency to allow all primigravidae to attempt vaginal delivery unless there is evidence of gross bony or fetal disease which would clearly prevent this.

There is now no place for assessment of pelvic capacity in early pregnancy. If the fetal head is engaged or can be made to engage in the pelvis at 36 weeks the likelihood of disproportion can be ruled out. The head will not be engaged at 36 weeks in almost a third of primigravidae and the majority of these will subsequently have normal deliveries. The reasons for a non-engaged head at 36 weeks are set out below, the first three being by far the commonest.

1. full rectum;
2. occipitoposterior position;
3. resistance from maternal soft parts (pelvic floor muscles and ligaments or thick lower uterine segment);
4. cephalopelvic disproportion;
5. placenta praevia;
6. increased pelvic tilt (high inclination brim) in African women;
7. polyhydramnios;
8. hydrocephalus;
9. brow presentation;
10. pelvic tumours.

If the head is deviated to one side and cannot be made to fit even partly into the pelvis the likelihood of placenta praevia is increased, and an ultrasonic scan for placental localization should be arranged forthwith. Otherwise it is reasonable for an experienced obstetrician to do a pelvic examination at this stage to exclude pelvic tumours and to make an assessment of the pelvic capacity. Unless a pelvic tumour is found or the size of the pelvis is clearly grossly reduced no further action is necessary until the onset of labour. If the head is still not engaged at the onset of labour, the labour is managed as a trial of labour.

Trial of Labour

A trial of labour is an attempt to achieve vaginal delivery in a case in which it is suspected that disproportion may exist. The patient is closely observed and is allowed to proceed in labour as long as good progress is maintained and no fetal distress develops, but otherwise Caesarean section is performed. Such labours should only be conducted in a major unit where Caesarean section is possible without delay. The conduct of trial of labour is described more fully in Chapter 14.

If on pelvic assessment at 36 weeks the obstetrician feels there is appreciable contraction he may order an X-ray pelvimetry. This is nowadays usually confined to a single erect lateral view because of the known risks to the fetus of antenatal radiography. On the basis of this pelvimetry the obstetrician may decide to do an elective Caesarean section, but in practice this is extremely rare. Following a Caesarean section for a failed trial of labour any subsequent delivery will be managed by elective Caesarean section.

Premature Labour

Any labour that occurs between 22 and 37 weeks should be considered a premature labour. Before 22 weeks there is no significant chance of the fetus surviving and after 37 weeks the risks are not significantly more than for a term fetus.

Causes of Premature Labour
These are:

1. incompetent cervix;
2. uterine abnormalities;
3. multiple pregnancy;
4. polyhydramnios;
5. premature rupture of membranes;
6. placental insufficiency;
7. fetal abnormalities;
8. antepartum haemorrhage;
9. intrauterine death;
10. uterine trauma;
11. maternal pyrexia or ill health (e.g. generalized infections or appendicitis);
12. premature labour is significantly more common in those of low socioeconomic class.

Management of Premature Labour
The patient should be admitted as quickly as possible to a major unit that has neonatal special care facilities. The baby is safer being transferred in utero than being delivered peripherally and then transferred in an incubator. If there is any possibility of imminent delivery a doctor or midwife should accompany the patient to hospital.

If the patient is seen early enough it may be possible to stop premature labour. It is generally advisable to try to stop premature labour unless the patient is beyond 36 weeks, but individual circumstances (for instance, the occurrence of haemorrhage or the suggestion of placental failure) will influence this decision. Labour may be arrested with the following types of drugs:

1. betasympathomimetic;
2. ethyl alcohol;
3. prostaglandin antagonists.

The drugs most widely used at present are the betasympathomimetic drugs salbutamol and ritodrine. These are given as an intravenous infusion, starting at a slow rate of infusion and increasing until the contractions stop or unacceptable side-effects are produced. A major side-effect with this treatment is maternal and fetal tachycardia. The maternal pulse should not be allowed to exceed 140 per minute. Additional side-effects that may be produced are hypotension, palpitations, tremor, anxiety and even panic attacks. With these drugs 80 per cent of premature labour can be arrested if the initial cervical dilatation is no more than 2 cm. When this intravenous regime is successful, long-term arrest may often be achieved with oral betasympathomimetic drugs.

There is now considerable evidence that surfactant production and functional lung maturity may be stimulated by high-dose steroid administration. A short course of dexamethasone given to the mother (4 mg 8 hourly for 48 hours) substantially reduces the likelihood of respiratory distress syndrome in the neonate. These dose levels of steroids should not be exceeded as there is some danger of actually encouraging premature labour.

Premature Rupture of Membranes

This is defined as rupture of the membranes before the onset of labour. It may occur at any stage of pregnancy up to or beyond term. Either the membranes lying over the internal cervical os may rupture (forewater rupture) or more commonly the leak occurs from the membranes higher up in the uterus (hindwater rupture). Forewater rupture is often due to an incompetent cervix which leaves an area of membrane unsupported and devitalized. With hindwater rupture a cause is rarely discovered. The risks of premature rupture of membranes are:

1. initiation of premature labour;
2. ascending infection (risk to mother as well as fetus);
3. cord prolapse (in labour, but rare before).

In addition, if delivery does not ensue and there is long-term leakage of liquor there is risk of producing fetal postural deformities (such as talipes). Of the first three risks cord prolapse is by far the rarest. In fact it is almost unknown before the onset of labour. The relative importance of the other two risks varies with the stage of pregnancy, but with modern management more babies are probably lost from prematurity than intrauterine infection.

Management of Premature Rupture of Membranes
In cases of doubt the diagnosis can usually be readily established by inserting a sterile vaginal speculum to see whether liquor is leaking through the cervix. This examination is important because many alleged premature ruptures of the membranes are in fact examples of urinary loss or imagination and patients may be unnecessarily admitted or even worse stimulated to deliver. If possible some liquor should be collected for culture and L/S ratio measurement.

Before 34 weeks aim to prolong the pregnancy.

1. Admit the patient to hospital for bed rest.
2. Avoid all vaginal examinations other than initial speculum examination to limit the risk of ascending infection.
3. Arrest premature labour if it occurs.
4. Consider elective delivery if the patient gets as far as 34 weeks or if there are any signs of ascending infection.
5. Antibiotics are not normally helpful unless there is evidence of infection.

After 34 weeks if the patient is in a unit with good neonatal facilities the balance of risks is probably in favour of delivery, particularly if a good L/S ratio has been found (but it is not always possible to obtain sufficient uncontaminated liquor for this to be done).

Delivery of Premature Infants
This is described in Chapter 14.

Placental Insufficiency – Intrauterine Growth Retardation
Placental insufficiency is now the major cause of perinatal death apart from fetal abnormalities. Placental insufficiency leads to fetal growth retardation in the early stages and fetal anoxia and death in more advanced stages. The main causes of placental insufficiency are as follows:

1. idiopathic;
2. multiple pregnancy;
3. smoking;
4. postmaturity;
5. antepartum haemorrhage;
6. essential hypertension;
7. other maternal illness (especially chronic urinary tract infection);
8. maternal malnutrition;
9. uterine infections (e.g. syphilis, cytomegalovirus);

10. it is also more common in women who have had previous small-for-dates babies, those of low socioecomomic class, primigravidae and women over 35 years of age.

Detection of Placental Insufficiency
Placental insufficiency should be anticipated in any of the abnormal situations listed above, but in a considerable proportion of cases there are no alerting factors in the woman's history. There are, however, clinical features of early placental failure which may be picked up by alert antenatal care as follows:

1. Uterine Size
With placental insufficiency the uterus appears small-for-dates. This is due partly to the fetus being small-for-dates and also to a considerably diminished volume of liquor (oligohydramnios). A small-for-dates uterus could also be due to wrong dates or fetal abnormality. Whenever the uterus is found to be small-for-dates, appropriate investigations should be instituted to determine which of these three factors is the cause.

2. Fetal Activity
Fetal activity will generally diminish when there is significant placental insufficiency. A number of units are now employing fetal activity charts (Kick Charts, or Count to Ten Charts), based on recent work from Cardiff. The woman is asked to note the time it takes for the fetus to move 10 times. This varies widely (from a few minutes to 12 hours), but anything over 12 hours is abnormal. These 'kick counts' can be done from 28 weeks on a weekly or a daily basis with minimal expense and inconvenience. They appear to offer a reliable method of picking up placental failure while there is still time to intervene.

3. Maternal Weight
Maternal weight should rise progressively through pregnancy, and failure to gain weight or loss of weight is frequently associated with placental failure. However, maternal weight is influenced by so many factors (e.g. sickness, oedema, diet) that it is not a very reliable sign.
   If any of these risk factors or clinical features suggest the possibility of placental failure, placental function tests must be arranged, and usually the patient will be admitted.

Placental Function Tests
1. Oestrogens
Either oestriol or total oestrogens may be measured in a 24-hour urine specimen or in a blood sample. These provide a reasonable indication of fetoplacental unit function. Repeated estimations to show a trend (which is normally upwards) give a more reliable indication of fetoplacental

function than isolated readings. Levels that fail to rise suggest placental insufficiency. Very low oestrogen levels will be found with intrauterine death, anencephaly, maternal high-dose steroid treatment, and the very rare placental sulphatase deficiency. Misleadingly low urinary oestrogen levels can be found during antibiotic treatment which interferes with one of the metabolic pathways in the mother, or with impaired renal function. Normal values are shown in Chapter 12.

2. Human Placental Lactogen
This is estimated on blood samples, and repeated readings are more reliable than isolated readings. Normal values are shown in Chapter 12.

3. Fetal Heart Rate Traces
The fetal heart rate may be recorded using a cardiotocograph machine with an external ultrasound transducer. The interpretation of these traces is comparable to the detection of fetal distress in labour (*see* Chapter 14).

4. Ultrasound Cephalometry
Serial ultrasound measurements of the fetal biparietal diameter or abdominal girth will give precise indications of fetal growth rate. Unfortunately the readings need to be at least a week apart to give significant results, so this method is of limited help in the relatively acute situation.

It is a mistake to rely on a single laboratory test, particularly if this is at variance with the clinical picture, but when placental function tests and clinical judgement together suggest that placental function is seriously impaired and intrauterine death is imminent the fetus must be delivered regardless of maturity.

ANTENATAL CARE – OTHER HIGH-RISK SITUATIONS
The Elderly Primigravida
Women who are pregnant for the first time at the age of 35 or more are known as elderly primigravidae. This is a term (like senile vaginitis) which may be offensive to the patient herself and should only be employed in a medical context.

The term is sometimes extended to those over 30 but there is no justification for this as the risks of pregnancy only increase appreciably over the age of 35. Age is a more important factor than nulliparity in determining the risk to the mother and fetus and indeed a 38-year-old woman having her fourth or fifth pregnancy is at greater risk than a 38-year-old primigravida. However, the elderly primigravida is considered a special case because the child is generally a particularly 'precious baby'. The woman will often have been infertile before conceiving and even if not her chances of conceiving again are less than those of a young woman. As general standards of antenatal and intrapartum care have improved there is no longer such a contrast between normal care and the special care of the

high-risk patient such as the elderly primigravida. However, most obstetricians agree that the elderly primigravida should:

1. be delivered in a specialist unit;
2. not be allowed to go appreciably past term;
3. have the fetus closely monitored in labour;
4. be delivered by Caesarean section at the first sign of any problems.

The Grand Multipara

A woman having her fifth or subsequent baby is known as a grand multipara and is at increased risk of perinatal mortality and serious maternal
problems. She will usually have had rapid, easy, normal deliveries previously.
She is often of low socioeconomic class and reluctant to accept obstetric
advice, particularly that she is likely to have any problems in this or
subsequent pregnancies. The main problems of these women of high
parity are:

1. chronic anaemia and malnutrition;
2. unstable lie, malpresentations and obstructed labour;
3. late engagement of the fetal head with the possibility of cord prolapse
   when the membranes rupture;
4. rapid labours, occasionally producing trauma to the baby by sudden
   compression and decompression of the head ('precipitate labour');
5. chronic anaemia.

The grand multiparous patient should be booked for a specialist
obstetric unit and should be followed closely in the antenatal period to
detect the problems listed above. Following delivery she should be offered
contraceptive advice in as subtle a way as possible, but she may well not
accept it.

The Obese Patient

The obese patient is at high risk for a number of reasons:

1. She is at increased risk of hypertension and pre-eclampsia.
2. Assessment of fetal, size, position and number is difficult or impossible.
3. The fetus also tends to be obese with increased risk of cephalopelvic disproportion and shoulder dystocia.
4 Anaesthesia and Caesarean section and other operative intervention
   are more difficult and also carry considerably increased risks.

Ideally the patient should be persuaded to lose weight before becoming
pregnant but this is rarely possible. If first seen when pregnant she should
be persuaded to maintain a diet which will result in minimal weight
increase during the pregnancy. She should be booked for a specialist unit

and followed closely in the antenatal period. A glucose tolerance test should be performed.

Rhesus Disease (Isoimmunization)

At the time of delivery or abortion (and occasionally at amniocentesis or external version) it is common for fetal blood cells to enter the maternal circulation. If the mother is rhesus-negative and the fetus rhesus-positive, these cells may sensitize her to produce anti-D rhesus antibodies. These antibodies are of the IgG series and in subsequent pregnancies can cross the placenta and affect the red cells of rhesus-positive fetuses. The red cells are haemolysed, producing fetal anaemia with increased bile pigment production. Most of this pigment is removed by the placenta (although some is excreted into the amniotic fluid) but following delivery the fetal liver is unable to cope with the increased haemolysis and jaundice develops rapidly – typically within a few hours of birth. The fetal anaemia may be severe enough to cause intrauterine death, which is usually preceded by the development in the fetus of gross oedema and ascites – a condition known as hydrops fetalis. In less severe cases the baby may be born alive, but then, if untreated, suffers deposits of bile pigment in the basal ganglia of the brain – a condition known as kernicterus, which can produce spasticity or death subsequently.

Nowadays rhesus disease is generally preventable, but previously about one-fifth of rhesus-negative women had developed rhesus antibodies by their second pregnancy and about a third of rhesus-negative women eventually did so. The severity of the disease tends to increase in successive pregnancies, but at a very variable rate, some women developing severe disease in their second pregnancy, while others develop only mild disease in spite of many pregnancies.

Prevention of Rhesus Disease

If anti-D immunoglobulin is given to the mother within 48 hours of delivery it coats any rhesus-positive cells in the maternal circulation, masks their antigenic sites and prevents sensitization. It is now routine to give 100 μg i.m. following delivery of a rhesus-positive baby to an unsensitized rhesus-negative mother. (If the mother is already sensitized such treatment has no value.) Maternal blood is also examined following delivery to judge the quantity of fetal cells in it, by the Kleihaur test. If large numbers of fetal cells are detected the dose of anti-D is increased correspondingly. Anti-D should also be given to unsensitized rhesus-negative women following: any abortion; external cephalic version; other significant uterine trauma and mismatched rhesus-positive blood transfusion.

If all these measures were employed universally rhesus disease would become rare, but many women abort without knowing their blood group or without telling their doctor, so that rhesus disease will not disappear in the foreseeable future.

Detection of Rhesus Disease

Every woman should be blood-grouped as early as possible in pregnancy and rhesus-negative women have tests for rhesus antibodies at booking, 28 weeks and 34 weeks.

Management of Rhesus Disease

Once rhesus antibodies are detected the woman is followed closely with regular antibody estimations (or titres). Low-level antibodies (less than 1·5 μg/ml) are generally associated with mild disease for which no active treatment is necessary, but higher serum antibody concentrations may be associated with moderate or severe disease, the actual severity being poorly

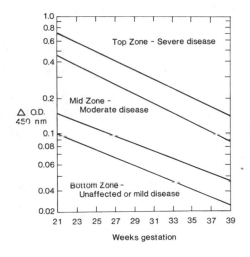

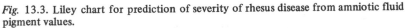

Fig. 13.3. Liley chart for prediction of severity of rhesus disease from amniotic fluid pigment values.

related to the antibody level. Examination of amniotic fluid obtained by amniocentesis gives a clearer guide to severity of the disease. The optical density of the amniotic fluid is calculated at 450 nm (the wavelength of bile pigment), and the results plotted on a Liley chart (*Fig.* 13.3). This gives zones for mild, moderate and severe disease for different stages of pregnancy. With severe disease the fetus is likely to die quickly in utero if not treated, whereas the fetus with moderate disease will generally survive until near term. Four forms of treatment are available antenatally:

1. Premature Delivery

If the fetus is past 34 weeks and the disease moderate to severe this may be the only treatment necessary.

2. *Intrauterine Transfusion*
The fetus may be transfused at intervals from 24 weeks with rhesus-negative cells – which will not be influenced by the maternal antibodies. This is achieved by introducing a catheter through a needle inserted through the maternal abdomen and uterine wall into the fetal abdominal cavity. Red cells are absorbed intact and enter the fetal circulation. This treatment is appropriate to those who are likely to have an intrauterine death before 34 weeks, and the fetal salvage rate is about 50 per cent.

3. *Plasmaphoresis*
Repeated plasmaphoresis can lower the maternal serum antibody concentration. This technique used in conjunction with intrauterine transfusion has extended the possibility of treatment to those with very severe disease.

4. *Phenobarbitone*
A dose of 100 mg daily (to the mother) for 2 weeks before elective delivery enhances fetal liver enzyme production promoting better bile pigment metabolism.
   Following delivery the affected child needs specialist neonatal paediatric care. The treatment employed includes exchange transfusions, top-up transfusions and light therapy.

Outlook for Future Pregnancies
It can be expected that any future rhesus-positive fetus will be at least as badly affected as in the last pregnancy, and probably worse. Whether the fetus will inevitably be affected depends on the rhesus group and zygosity of the father, so paternal rhesus genotyping is normally carried out in cases of rhesus disease. If the father is heterozygous rhesus-positive (Dd) there is a 50 per cent chance of his child being rhesus-negative, whereas a homozygous (DD) father can only produce rhesus-positive children.

MEDICAL ABNORMALITIES COMPLICATING PREGNANCY

The more important medical disorders of pregnancy will be considered here. For fuller accounts of this fascinating area of medicine the reader is referred to the book list at the end of this chapter.

Non Pre-eclamptic Hypertension

Pregnancy presents a good opportunity for screening for chronic hypertensive states. Essential hypertension occurs in about 1 per cent of pregnancies, and other forms of non pre-eclamptic hypertension very much more rarely. Patients with blood pressure of more than 140/90 in early pregnancy should be admitted for tests and observation. The patient should undergo a thorough general examination with palpation of femoral and radial pulses to exclude coarctation, auscultation of renal arteries to exclude renal artery stenosis and assessment of cardiac size and normality.

The tests should include renal function tests, repeated midstream urine cultures and estimation of urinary catecholamines or VMA (vanillylmandelic acid) to exclude a phaeochromocytoma. The observation of the trend in blood pressure over the course of a few days gives a good indication of its true level and of the prognosis for the pregnancy, a fall in blood pressure with rest being a good sign.

Essential hypertension approximately doubles the perinatal mortality overall, but minor degrees of essential hypertension with a diastolic of less than 100 mm of mercury carry virtually no risk. With the more severe degrees the mother is also at risk of placental abruption, and of cerebral vascular accident, heart failure and possible permanent deterioration of hypertension if there is superadded eclampsia. The risk to mother and fetus is very much more if there is albuminuria present in the first half of pregnancy or if superadded pre-eclampsia develops later.

Essential hypertension of a more than minor degree is probably best managed in conjunction with a physician, If hypotensive treatment is necessary this is ideally best started before the patient embarks on the pregnancy. In pregnancy hypotensive treatment is probably beneficial if the average blood pressure exceeds 150/100. The hypotensive most often used is methyldopa. Extra rest limits blood pressure rise and improves placental perfusion, and the more severe cases may need to be admitted to hospital for most of the pregnancy. A close watch on placental function and fetal growth rate is necessary, and premature induction may well offer the best chance to the fetus. Ergometrine should be avoided at the time of delivery.

Phaeochromocytoma

This is a very rare but extremely serious complication of pregnancy. The maternal mortality rate of the published cases exceeds 50 per cent, and was 100 per cent where a hypertensive crisis occurred in labour. A phaeochromocytoma should be suspected if hypertension is severe or intermittent, and appropriate biochemical tests should be carried out. If a phaeochromocytoma is discovered it is best removed without delay and before delivery.

Diabetes in Pregnancy

Diabetes has become a more common complication of pregnancy as better control has led to improved fertility. Maternal diabetes carries very considerable potential hazards to both mother and fetus; great care is needed to detect all cases of diabetes in pregnancy, and great skill is needed to minimize those risks.

Effect of Pregnancy on Diabetes

1. Insulin requirements generally increase appreciably and control becomes more difficult.

2. Glycosuria is no longer a reliable indication of degree of diabetic control.
3. Some women who had normal glucose tolerance before pregnancy will develop chemical or clinical diabetes in pregnancy (often reverting to normal after delivery).

Effect of Diabetes in Pregnancy
1. Without meticulous diabetic control the fetus grows abnormally rapidly, with increased fat deposition. This leads to an increased likelihood of mechanical problems at delivery.
2. Without meticulous control there is a high incidence of intrauterine death in the last months of pregnancy.
3. There is an increased incidence of polyhydramnios, especially if diabetic control is poor.
4. The incidence of fetal abnormality is increased.
5. The neonate is at increased risk of serious problems, including respiratory distress syndrome (RDS) and hypoglycaemia.

Detection of Diabetes in Pregnancy
Glucose tolerance tests should be done in the first half of pregnancy in the following circumstances for women not previously known to be diabetic.

1. Close family history of diabetes.
2. Glycosuria on two occasions during pregnancy or heavy (2·0 per cent) glycosuria on one occasion.
3. Any previous baby weighing over 9 lb. (4·2 kg).
4. Previous unexplained stillbirth.
5. Marked obesity.

This screening of at-risk cases is particularly important since the risks run by an undiagnosed early diabetic far exceed those of a well-managed established diabetic.

Management of Diabetes in Pregnancy
Management of the pregnant diabetic is difficult and is best carried out by teams with a particular interest in this field draining all the cases in the area. The key principles are summarized here:

1. Care should be shared between an obstetrician and a physician specializing in diabetes, preferably seeing the patient together.
2. Insulin requirements increase in pregnancy and most patients need a twice-daily injection of both short- and long-acting insulins to maintain good control. If the patient is not already on this sort of regime it is usual to admit her at about 12 weeks for the change over.
3. Control is judged on the basis of blood sugar levels, and not on the degree of glycosuria.

4. Tight diabetic control reduces the incidence of pregnancy complications, so blood sugars should be kept within the normal non-
diabetic range. A 'blood sugar run' consisting of 3 preprandial
samples and 1 late-night sample is taken at intervals during the
pregnancy, corresponding to the frequency of normal antenatal care
(i.e. monthly initially, reducing to weekly in late pregnancy). These
samples should all contain less than 5·5 mmol/l (100 mg per cent)
glucose. Estimation of the maternal glycosylated haemoglobin levels
(HbA_1) gives a good idea of the level of control over the past few
weeks.

5. Any obstetric complication or general ill health (particularly infections) are treated very seriously and generally merit admission.

6. Fetoplacental function is monitored closely in the last trimester.

7. The patient is delivered at about 38 weeks, either by inducing labour
if the obstetric situation is favourable or by elective Caesarean
section if there are any complications at all.

8. The fetus is monitored in labour, and early recourse is made to
Caesarean section if good progress is not maintained, or at any
suspicion of fetal distress.

9. An experienced neonatal paediatrician should attend the delivery.

Heart Disease in Pregnancy

Heart disease in pregnancy is now relatively rare and is found in only 1 or
2 per 1000 pregnancies, with congenital heart disease being more common
than rheumatic heart disease. The haemodynamic changes of pregnancy
and delivery throw extra strain on the heart (Chapter 12) and result in
increased risk to the cardiac patient. There were 20 deaths in England and
Wales in the years 1973–75 attributable to heart disease in pregnancy.

The following are the main effects of pregnancy on the patient with
heart disease.

1. *Increased functional disability.* Pregnancy frequently results in a
slight worsening of the functional disability.

2. *Risk of heart failure.* There is increased risk of both congestive
failure and pulmonary oedema. Respiratory infection may precipitate congestive failure, and pulmonary oedema is particularly
likely in patients with tight mitral stenosis and an efficient myo-
cardium.

3. *Risk of endocarditis.* Bacterial endocarditis is a rare but definite
complication of delivery.

Management of Heart Disease in Pregnancy

1. Seek the advice of a cardiologist early in pregnancy, and unless the
disease is trivial manage the patient jointly throughout pregnancy.

2. Termination is not indicated and must be avoided until failure is

controlled. It may then be carried out for the usual (non-cardiac) reasons.

3. Advise extra rest. The more serious cases will be admitted to hospital for a period of rest before delivery, and any patient developing heart failure will need admission for the whole pregnancy.
4. Treat respiratory infection and anaemia vigorously.
5. Allow spontaneous labour and vaginal delivery unless there are obstetric contraindications.
6. Prophylactic antibiotics (ampicillin, gentamycin) during labour.
7. In the more serious cases perform elective forceps delivery.
8. Avoid ergometrine or other oxytocics in those at risk of pulmonary oedema.

Liver Disease in Pregnancy

Jaundice

Jaundice is a rare but potentially very serious complication of pregnancy. It may be classified into (1) jaundice peculiar to pregnancy and (2) jaundice incidental to pregnancy.

Jaundice Peculiar to Pregnancy
1. Acute fatty liver of pregnancy.
2. Recurrent intrahepatic cholestatic jaundice.
3. Jaundice complicating severe pre-eclampsia.
4. Jaundice complicating hyperemesis.

Acute fatty liver of pregnancy is a rare condition usually occurring in the last weeks of pregnancy. It is characterized by rapidly progressive jaundice, abdominal pain and vomiting, clotting disorders, fetal death and usually maternal coma and death. Its aetiology is thought to be linked to the breakdown of protein synthesis in the liver under the increased demands of pregnancy, and of the reported cases in recent years most have been associated with the use of parenteral tetracyclines. If the patient is to have any prospect of survival she is best treated in a specialist liver unit.

Recurrent intrahepatic cholestatic jaundice is relatively more common. It is also known as benign idiopathic jaundice of pregnancy and gestational hepatosis. It is characterized by a mild jaundice occurring in late pregnancy, often associated with marked generalized pruritus. It tends to recur in subsequent pregnancies, and also possibly if the patient takes oral contraceptives. A raised alkaline phosphatase and a mildly raised bilirubin are the common biochemical findings. It has previously been thought that the condition does not affect the outcome of pregnancy, but recent reports suggest a mild increase in perinatal mortality and postpartum haemorrhage.

Jaundice is a rare complication of either severe pre-eclampsia, or eclampsia, or hyperemesis. The proper and prompt management of the underlying condition should, however, prevent either the development of jaundice or its progression.

Incidental Jaundice in Pregnancy
All forms of jaundice may occur in pregnancy, viral hepatitis and gallstones being the commonest causes. The viruses of both infectious hepatitis and serum hepatitis will cross the placenta, and special precautions are necessary in handling infected patients, particularly at the time of delivery, to avoid the transmission of infection to the obstetrician or midwife.

Pregnancy in a well-nourished population in general has little effect on the course of incidental liver disease. The biochemical disturbances of liver disease do, however, seem to increase appreciably the risk of stillbirth, to interfere with uterine contractility and to lead to clotting failure, so that specialist medical and obstetric care is vital in all cases of liver disease in pregnancy.

Thyroid Disease in Pregnancy
The changes in thyroid physiology in pregnancy (see Chapter 12) make assessment of thyroid function somewhat more difficult in pregnancy. Binding proteins, including thyroid binding globulin, increase in concentration in response to oestrogen, so that protein bound iodine rises to well above non-pregnant levels. Also pulse rate and basal metabolic rate increase. However, the blood levels of the free hormones, thyroxine, tri-iodothyronine and thyroid-stimulating hormone should remain unchanged, and departures from the normal range indicate thyroid disease.

Thyrotoxicosis
Untreated thyrotoxicosis tends to reduce fertility, and if it does occur in pregnancy it increases the rate of abortion, pre-eclampsia, premature labour and perinatal mortality. Thyrotoxicosis is generally treated medically during pregnancy with carbimazole. If the mother is maintained meticulously at euthyroid levels, there is probably no excess risk to the fetus, but accidental overdose with carbimazole (or any of the other antithyroid drugs, all of which cross the placenta) may render the fetus hypothyroid, with goitre formation or cretinism in extreme cases. Some physicians guard against this possibility by giving 1-thyroxine 0·3 mg daily as well as carbimazole. Radioiodine should not be used either diagnostically or therapeutically in pregnancy because of the risk of long-term fetal thyroid damage.

Hypothyroidism
Hypothyroidism also impairs fertility and is rarely found in pregnancy. If untreated or inadequately treated there is increased risk of abortion, fetal abnormality and stillbirth. Treatment with thyroxine should be instituted

gradually, and should aim to render the patient euthyroid. Patients already being treated before pregnancy for hypothyroidism are likely to need increased doses of thyroxine.

Urinary Tract Disease in Pregnancy

Asymptomatic Bacteriuria

About 6 per cent of pregnant women have asymptomatic bacteriuria, which is defined as more than 100 000 organisms per ml in freshly voided urine. The composition of the bacteriuric population is not constant, with some women spontaneously clearing their urinary tract of significant bacteriuria, while others have permanent bacteriuria often related to underlying renal infection. Bacteriuria has been associated with:

1. increased likelihood of developing acute pyelonephritis in pregnancy;
2. increased rate of premature delivery;
3. decreased mean birth weight;
4. anaemia.

Bacteriuria is more common in lower social classes, and this association may account for all the factors above, apart from the increased risk of pyelonephritis. It is a routine in most clinics now to screen at booking for asymptomatic bacteriuria. Those with positive tests are treated with a 7-day course of ampicillin or sulphonamides, which will cure about 75 per cent. Those who get recurrent bacteriuria are treated again, and any who subsequently relapse merit full renal investigation following pregnancy as they are likely to have chronic pyelonephritis or serious renal tract abnormalities.

Acute Pyelonephritis

Acute pyelonephritis is more common in pregnancy because of the relative stasis in the urinary tract brought about by the dilatation of ureters and renal calyces, and because of the increased sugar content of pregnancy urine. About half of acute pyelonephritis arises in those with asymptomatic bacteriuria. The disease may present in a mild form with little more than nausea and malaise, or in a severe form with high pyrexia, rigors, vomiting, loin pain and tenderness, and dysuria. The more serious forms may lead to premature labour and occasionally to intrauterine death of the fetus (due to the high pyrexia). Permanent renal damage may also follow if treatment is not promptly instituted. The diagnosis is usually made without difficulty and can be confirmed by urine examination. The causative organism is nearly always *E.coli.* Treatment should be started without waiting for culture results. It is important to avoid high pyrexia by tepid sponging or by giving aspirin. Anaemia is a common sequel, presumably due to suppression of erythropoetin production from the kidney.

Chronic Pyelonephritis and Chronic Nephritis

These two conditions often present in the same way in pregnancy with evidence of renal impairment, possibly with albuminuria or hypertension, but without clear evidence of infection or of a nephritic origin for the impaired renal function. They may only be distinguishable by renal biopsy which is rarely used in pregnancy. They may have a very serious effect on the course of pregnancy, increasing the likelihood of early and middle trimester abortion, of intrauterine growth retardation and of superadded pre-eclampsia. The outlook is correspondingly worse where there is:

1. albuminuria;
2. hypertension;
3. blood urea raised above 9 mmol/litre (50 mg per cent).

Differention from pre-eclampsia may present some difficulty if the patient is not seen in the first half of pregnancy; otherwise investigation as outlined on p. 204 for non pre-eclamptic hypertension will usually give a sufficiently clear diagnosis to allow the pregnancy to be managed satisfactorily. Consideration should be given to terminating the pregnancy in the more serious cases of renal impairment. In less severe cases, close antenatal care, treatment of infection, placental function monitoring and extra rest will generally allow a successful outcome.

Acute Nephritis and Renal Tuberculosis

Both of these conditions are now very rare complications of pregnancy, and their general management is little affected by the coexistence of the pregnancy.

Anaemia in Pregnancy

Some degree of anaemia is very common in pregnancy. The significant increase in maternal blood volume (+ 30 per cent) and the ability of the placenta to extract iron from the maternal circulation to meet its own needs (150 mg) and those of the fetus (400–450 mg) mean that a considerable demand is put on the maternal iron stores. Many women, and particularly those of lower socioeconomic classes, will have depleted iron stores at the beginning of pregnancy, and cannot expect to absorb the required quantity of iron (3–4 mg per day) from their normal diet. In such circumstances iron deficiency anaemia develops. The 1958 Perinatal Mortality Survey showed that severe anaemia (haemoglobin below 8·9 g per 100 ml) was associated with a twofold increase in perinatal mortality. While it can be argued that some of the excess risk is related to the poor socioeconomic conditions which were responsible for the anaemia, there can be little doubt that severe anaemia directly increases the risk to both mother and fetus. It has become a widespread routine in this and other countries to give the pregnant woman prophylactic iron and folic acid supplements from 12 weeks onwards. Iron should be avoided in early pregnancy because there is some evidence of a tendency to increased fetal abnormality rates. A single daily dose of one of the proprietary sustained release preparations such as Pregaday, Fefol or Slow Fe-folic is suitable. Iron preparations tend to produce constipation and make the motions a very dark colour.

Much the most common cause of anaemia in this country is iron deficiency, generally related to failure to take iron supplements. Iron deficiency may, however, also be due to chronic infection (particularly urinary tract infection) and to chronic blood loss (piles, intestinal neoplasia, etc.). Haemoglobinopathies are common in Negroid patients, and thalassaemias are common in those with Mediterranean ancestry. In immigrants, hookworm infestation, malaria and other parasites are possibilities. Folic acid deficiency is particularly likely with multiple pregnancy.

Investigation and Treatment of Anaemia in Pregnancy
Immigrant populations will normally be screened for abnormal haemoglobins at booking. Otherwise the initial investigation of anaemia will usually be a full blood count and film. If these show a picture of iron deficiency it is usually sufficient to treat the anaemia with oral iron and folic acid without further investigation. If the patient fails to respond to this treatment it is appropriate to do further investigations as follows:

    serum iron concentration;
    iron binding capacity;
    serum folate concentration;
    serum vitamin B_{12} concentration;
    examination of stool for occult blood and parasites;
    urine culture.

If these investigations reveal nothing other than iron deficiency due to the patient's unwillingness or inability to take oral iron it may be appropriate to treat her with parenteral iron. Neither intravenous nor intramuscular iron preparations should be used lightly as both can produce unpleasant side-effects — anaphylactic reactions with intravenous iron and very unsightly skin staining with intramuscular preparations. It is probably unnecessary to treat anaemia in this way unless the haemoglobin is below 9 g per 100 ml. Very occasionally with severe anaemia it may be advisable to transfuse blood before labour, and in extreme cases this should be done by exchange transfusions or by combining intravenous frusemide with transfusion to avoid the hazards of heart failure.

In cases of haemoglobinopathy iron stores may be overloaded in spite of anaemia, and increased iron administration may be unnecessary and even hazardous. The detailed management of haemoglobinopathies in pregnancy falls outside the scope of this book, but detailed accounts of their management may be found in the books mentioned below.

Further Reading
Barnes C. G. (1979) *Medical Disorders in Obstetric Practice*, 4th ed. Oxford, Blackwell.
McClure Browne J. C. and Dixon G. (ed.) (1978) *Browne's Antenatal Care*, 11th ed. Edinburgh, Churchill Livingstone.
Scott J. S. and Jones W. R. (ed.) (1976) *Immunology of Human Reproduction*. London, Academic.
Stevenson A. C. and Davison B. C. C. (1976) *Genetic Counselling*. London, Heinemann.

Chapter fourteen

Intrapartum Care

Perhaps no field of medicine, certainly of obstetrics, has seen as many technological advances in so few years as intrapartum care, especially that of the fetus. With rising socioeconomic standards the general health of mothers has improved greatly, and obstetrical hazards such as rickets are now virtually a thing of the past in the UK obstetric population.

New methods of monitoring have made labour less hazardous for mother and fetus, with the emphasis on prevention rather than treatment of disaster. The delivery suite is to be regarded as an intensive care unit, and unexplained intrapartum fetal death should not occur. It has been claimed that total intrapartum monitoring of the fetus would reduce the Caesarean section rate and reduce intrapartum fetal mortality and morbidity, but the financial implications of fetal monitoring in labour are enormous. There are many questions as yet unanswered. Should total monitoring be the aim? Certainly at present the equipment involved is distasteful to many patients and, for some, downright unacceptable. Labour is a physiological progress which if left to its own devices is associated with a maternal and fetal mortality and morbidity rate. It may be regarded as a natural mechanism for controlling population. Groups favouring a return to natural childbirth and home delivery in, for example, California, have experienced an increase in maternal and infant death. It may be a mother's right to choose where she is going to have her child, but that·choice should be made in the knowledge of the facts. Also she is making a choice for her child – does she have the right to do this? A damaged child is a financial burden to the State as well as a burden to its parents. With the emphasis on more acceptable methods of monitoring, the humanizing of hospital and early discharge to home, increasing numbers of mothers are happy to have their babies in major obstetric units appreciating the safety and the expertise available for both mother and infant should a problem occur.

NORMAL LABOUR
Management of Normal Labour
Preparation for labour starts in the antenatal period and should be directed towards the mother's mental and physical state and should include the

father if they both wish. With confidence in herself and her attendants, and supported by her husband in familiar pleasant surroundings, a woman's labour can be an interesting and rewarding experience. The sterile, hostile delivery rooms of old have been replaced in many places by rooms with attractive screens, pictures, radio and often television. The patient will have visited these rooms during her parentcraft classes. Education about the onset, stages and mechanism of labour is as important to the mother as it is to the medical student and pupil midwife.

The Onset of Labour

The initial diagnosis of the onset of labour is made by the patient, who then presents herself for admission to her place of confinement, which for most women in the UK is a maternity hosiptal. The diagnosis has to be confirmed, as the patient, especially if she is a primigravida, may be mistaken. The onset of labour is heralded by one or more of the following: contractions, 'a show' or the 'waters breaking'. Since uterine contractions are noticed during late pregnancy a frequency of one contraction every 10 minutes (1 in 10) is a practical guide to the uterine contractions of labour. The difference between the contractions of late pregnancy and the contractions of labour is that the latter dilate the cervix. The onset of painful regular contractions may be accompanied by a 'show', that is the loss vaginally of the mucus plug in the cervix. This mucus is often streaked with blood. The membranes usually rupture fairly late in labour but occasionally may be the first sign of labour. They may cause a major flood and considerable inconvenience, or leak in a dribbling fashion.

On admission, after history taking and examination the patient is requested to take a bath. There is no point in shaving the pubic hair unless Caesarean section is contemplated and an enema is only necessary if the patient is constipated. The patient and her husband, if they both wish, are then conducted to the delivery suite. If there is a first stage sitting room and she is in early labour, she and her husband may spend the initial part of labour here, repairing to the delivery room later, but the construction of the delivery unit dictates management of the first stage to some extent.

Mechanism of Labour

This term is used to describe the movements of the fetal head and trunk through the maternal pelvis. These have been outlined in Chapter 2. The head enters the true pelvis before or during labour and usually engages in the transverse diameter, i.e. the sagittal suture of the fetal skull is at right angles to the anteroposterio. diameter of the maternal pelvis. With contractions the head descends and becomes more flexed. Thus the occiput becomes the lowest part of the head as a result of flexion and reaches the pelvic floor first. Here the levator ani muscles meet in the midline and form a gutter channelling downwards and forwards. The uterine contractions and tone in the levators act together on the head to produce internal rotation (that is the occiput is rotated forwards so that it comes to lie beneath the symphysis pubis). Further descent occurs, the occiput escapes from under the pubic arch, and the head is born by extension, When the widest diameter comes through the introitus the head is said to crown (*see Fig.* 14.1). As the head is born, the shoulders enter the pelvis. They pass

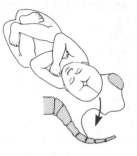 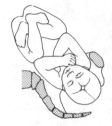

a. Head enters the true pelvis   b. Head descends to pelvic floor

Fig. 14.1. Mechanism of labour.

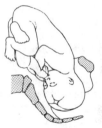 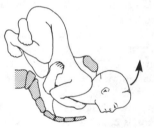

c. Internal rotation, occiput comes   d. Further descent, head is born
   to lie beneath symphysis pubis   by extension

through the widest diameter of the pelvic inlet and rotate to accommodate themselves to the widest diameter of the outlet, that is the anteroposterior (AP) diameter. As the shoulders rotate into the AP diameter, the delivered head is carried round 90°. This external rotation (or restitution) is readily seen. The anterior shoulder escapes from under the symphysis and the trunk is born by lateral flexion.

The Stages of Labour

Three stages of labour are recognized.

Stage 1 is from the onset of labour to full dilatation of the cervical os. This usually lasts between 8 and 10 hours in the primigravida and 6 and 8 hours in the multigravida. During this stage the head descends and becomes flexed.

Stage 2 is from full dilatation to birth of the fetus. This usually lasts between 40 and 60 minutes in the primigravida and 10 to 15 minutes in the multigravida. The second stage may be divided into two phases. During the first phase the vagina dilates, allowing further descent of the head to the pelvic floor where internal rotation occurs. With the second phase, further descent occurs, the occiput reaches the perineum and escapes from under the pubic arch and the head is born. This concept of two phases to the second stage originates from Dublin and is of particular relevance when considering forceps delivery (*see below*).
Stage 3 is from the birth of the fetus to the delivery of the placenta and membranes.

Maternal Wellbeing

The indices of maternal wellbeing are: mental state, physical condition and progress.

The importance of the mother's mental state must never be overlooked since terror and hysteria can have an adverse affect on the progress of labour and overbreathing leads to tetany, respiratory alkalosis and impaired fetal oxygenation. The electrolyte imbalance may cause uterine contractions to become inefficient. The husband can give support and comfort and his presence is to be encouraged if he and his wife so wish. Neither should be made to feel guilty, however, if the husband's presence is not desired.

The mother's physical condition is assessed very frequently, with particular attention to blood pressure, pulse, temperature and hydration. Bland fluids are to be encouraged but all food avoided, and an oral liquid antacid is taken every 2 hours in case a general anaesthetic is required. The patient is encouraged to empty her bladder at frequent intervals, and the volume of each specimen is measured and recorded. Each specimen is tested for albumin, ketones and sugar. Dehydration and ketosis can be prevented or treated by an intravenous dextrose infusion but this will only be necessary if labour is relatively long.

During labour the patient should adopt whatever posture she desires. She should be encouraged to be as free as possible to walk, stand, sit or lie at will, but her wishes may be hampered by intravenous infusions, monitoring systems and the need to carry out observations. She should not lie flat on her back since pressure from the gravid uterus on the inferior vena cava will cause supine hypotension and diminished uterine and placental perfusion. Labour is a painful process for the majority of women and although psychoprophylaxis, hypnosis and acupuncture may prevent or relieve pain, the majority of women require analgesia. The type and timing of analgesia is crucial and individual.

Pain Relief
Pethidine 50 to 100 mg intramuscularly is widely used in the first stage of labour. The State Registered midwife is allowed to prescribe up to 2

doses of 100 mg of pethidine. The dose should be given with thought to the patient's physique, and it should not be given within 4 hours of delivery — if such a judgement is possible — since it depresses the neonatal respiratory centre. It may cause vomiting. Mild analgesics like aspirin have no place since they are not effective. Strong analgesics like morphine and Omnopon cause such profound neonatal respiratory depression that they are generally avoided.

Epidural anaesthesia produces total pain relief without impairment of consciousness or fetal depression, but by relaxing levator tone interferes with the mechanism of labour, particularly at the stage of internal rotation, and makes maternal voluntary expulsive efforts difficult, thus increasing the incidence of malrotation and forceps delivery.

Entonox (nitrous oxide 50 per cent, oxygen 50 per cent) is an inhalational analgesic especially effective at the end of the first stage and during the second stage since it is absorbed and expelled very rapidly. Inhalation should begin just before the contraction starts and before the patient feels pain, for it takes 15–20 seconds to work. Timing the contractions is a prerequisite for this form of analgesia to be effective.

Progress of Labour
Dilatation of the cervix can be assessed by vaginal examination and should occur at the rate of 1 cm or more per hour once labour is well established. All vaginal examinations must be carried out with the utmost respect for strict asepsis whether or not the membranes have ruptured. Abdominal palpation of the fetal head reveals descent of the head and it is currently customary to divide the head into fifths and record the number of fifths palpable: for instance, when all the head is palpable above the pelvic brim it is recorded as five fifths (5/5) and when none of the head is palpable, no fifths (0/5). Descent of the head can also be judged on vaginal examination by estimating the distance of the lowest part of the fetal head above or below the level of the ischial spines: for instance, if the head is 3 cm above the ischial spines this is recorded as minus 3 (−3), if the head is palpable 2 cm below the level of the ischial spines it is recorded as plus 2 (+2). As the head descends through the pelvis there is usually a degree of moulding, that is the skull bones overlap. If there is any delay in descent, caput forms, that is the scalp becomes oedematous and thickened making palpation of the sutures and fontanelles difficult. One must beware of considering caput as a reference point when defining the descent of the head since the thickened oedematous scalp may mislead one into thinking that the head is lower in the pelvis than it really is. Progress in labour is further monitored by the strength and frequency of uterine contractions, and these are recorded by one of the following methods:

1. Palpation. This is a subjective and variable observation requiring experience for reliability but is of no inconvenience to the patient.

2. An external pressure transducer may be strapped to the anterior abdominal wall measuring contractions more accurately, although movement and anterior abdominal wall fat may make recording difficult. It is somewhat inhibiting for the patient since she has to remain attached to the recorder.

3. Internal uterine pressure may be measured via a catheter introduced into the uterus after rupture of the membranes. This may be a fluid-filled open-ended catheter or a solid catheter. The first type of catheter is connected to a pressure transducer, the second type has a transducer in its tip. Although intrauterine pressure may be measured precisely, this method is invasive and carries the risk of infection and placental damage. It also requires the patient to remain in close contact with the recorder unless a telemetric system is being used. In telemetry the transducer is attached to a transmitter strapped to the patient's thigh and radio signals of intrauterine pressure are sent to a receiver, and thus the patient is able to be mobile while recordings are being made.

Fetal Wellbeing

Labour is a hazardous time to any fetus since with each contraction blood flow through the intervillous space ceases and the oxygen supply to the fetus is reduced. A normal fetus can accommodate to these intermittent periods of hypoxia for some time, but an already hypoxic fetus is in jeopardy. Consequently careful monitoring of fetal wellbeing in labour is necessary.

Indices of fetal wellbeing are fetal heart rate, meconium, and fetal blood pH.

Fetal Heart Rate

The fetal heart may be observed in various ways.

1. Auscultation with a Pinard fetal stethoscope through the mother's anterior abdominal wall is the most widely used method (originally described by Lannaec of Brittany). It is most informative if auscultation is continued through and after a contraction so that alterations in rate can be appreciated. If no contractions occur then auscultation over at least 2 minutes and during fetal movements is valuable.

2. Ultrasound. The alterations of blood flow in the fetal heart can be detected by the Doppler effect. This signal can be obtained through the mother's anterior abdominal wall.

3. Electrocardiography picks up the electrical activity of the fetal heart with a clip attached directly to the fetal scalp.

The terms used in the study of continuous fetal heart traces are shown in *Fig.* 14.2.

The following fetal heart rate features are potential signs of fetal distress.

1. A fetal heart rate above 160 or below 120 per minute.
2. Lack of beat to beat variation (minor variations in heart rate which occur in response to autonomic reflex activity).
3. Slowing in heart rate occurring during or immediately after contractions (dips and decelerations, *see Fig.* 14.3).

Less than 50 per cent of cases with these heart rate changes will have true fetal distress.

Meconium

The fetal gut may contract and the anal sphincter relax under hypoxic conditions, releasing meconium into the amniotic fluid. The presence of meconium staining in the liquor is, however, an unreliable sign of fetal distress on its own. If the fetal heart rate is normal then about 10 per cent of patients with meconium-stained liquor have a distressed fetus, but if the fetal heart rate is abnormal the figure is about 20 per cent. In order that this sign is not missed, amniotomy (rupture of the membranes) is now a routine practice once labour is established, that is the cervix is dilating at the rate of 1 cm or more per hour and is at least 3 cm dilated.

Fetal Blood pH

If hypoxia is present, carbon dioxide and lactic acid accumulate and the pH of the blood falls below 7·2. If hypoxia is suspected because of meconium or dips (slowing) in the fetal heart trace, a fetal blood sample may be taken to confirm hypoxia. An amnioscope is passed through the cervix and the fetal skull visualized. The scalp is stabbed with a very short protected blade and blood is drawn up into an heparinized tube for pH analysis. The pH in the first stage falls but normally remains above 7·25. In the second stage of normal labour· the pH occasionally falls to 7·15. A maternal acidosis may cause the fetal pH to fall, and correction of the maternal acidosis with bicarbonate will raise the fetal pH. If the fetal pH falls below 7·2 for whatever reason the fetus must be delivered at once as fetal death is imminent.

The Partograph

This is a visual display of the indices of maternal and fetal wellbeing mentioned above, together with progress displayed as cervical dilatation and descent of the head on abdominal palpation. Such charts have proved useful in the early detection of abnormal labour. Whether partographs are used or not, regular recordings of maternal and fetal wellbeing and progress are essential during the first stage of labour.

Active and Accelerated Labour

These terms have unfortunately caused much confusion with the public. If labour is not progressing normally, i.e. the cervix is not dilating at the usual rate of 1 cm or more per hour, then in order to prevent a prolonged

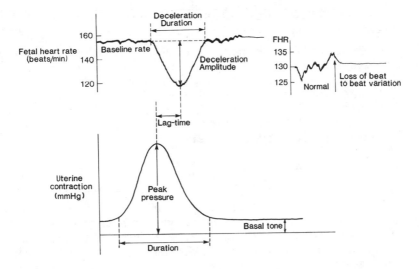

Fig. 14.2. Terms used in the study of continuous fetal heart traces.

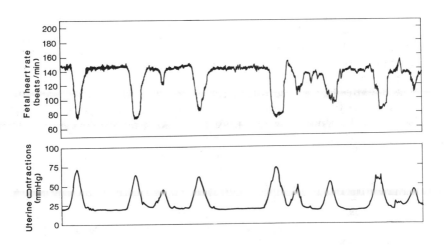

Fig. 14.3. Dips and decelerations.

labour, with all its attendant maternal and fetal problems, steps are taken to normalize the rate of cervical dilatation.

1. Rupture of the membranes accompanied by stretching of the cervix and lower segment will stimulate uterine contractions, probably by releasing prostaglandins, and improve cervical dilatation.
2. Intravenous syntocinon infusion will improve the strength and frequency of uterine contractions, especially if the membranes are ruptured, and efficient uterine contractions are necessary for delivery.

These two steps may be taken at the same time.

The Second Stage

Phase 1 of the second stage may go unheralded since during this time the patient has no desire to push. Although the cervix is fully dilated the vagina has to dilate and uterine contractions have to bring the head to the pelvic floor. When the head reaches the pelvic floor and internal rotation occurs the patient usually has an overwhelming desire to push. Involuntary expulsive efforts are seen and there is evidence accruing that the patient should be encouraged to push as she feels the need to, rather than the traditional long-sustained pushing with each contraction. With each expulsive effort the head further descends bulging the perineum and causing the anus to pout. Internal rotation may be seen to occur on the perineum. Inhalational analgesia, if analgesia is required, is ideal during the second stage and should be inhaled before the contraction starts, as indicated previously.

The fetal heart rate must be recorded after each contraction if a continuous record is not available. During the second stage, and especially at delivery, strict asepsis must be practised. The bladder must be empty and the membranes ruptured with Kocher's forceps if they have not already ruptured. Delivery usually takes place with the patient in a semi-sitting position, although some patients prefer the left lateral position. The patient should be allowed to adopt whatever position she wishes provided that the attendant is able to control the delivery of the head and have access to the face, eyes, nose and mouth of the fetus at once, and be able to protect the perineum from tearing. If it looks as though the perineum is going to tear, an episiotomy (*see below*) is carried out. After crowning, the head is delivered slowly by extension. The baby's pharynx should be cleared with a mucus aspirator during restitution and before the delivery of the shoulders. The baby's head is then drawn towards the mother's sacrum, aiding the passage of the anterior shoulder under the symphysis. The head is then drawn up towards the symphysis and the posterior shoulder slides over the perineum. Gentle traction with one finger in the posterior axilla may be necessary.

As the trunk delivers, the baby is taken up on to the mother's abdomen so that she may see and feel and hold the baby at once if this is feasible.

The cord is clamped and cut at least 5 cm from the umbilicus. The baby must not be allowed to get cold and must, therefore, be wrapped, The baby may need further mucus aspiration, but there is no reason why, if its condition is satisfactory, the wrapping and aspiration should not be done in the mother's arms.

The Third Stage

Active management of the third stage is usual today. An oxytocic, usually syntometrine 1 ampoule (containing ergometrine 0·5 mg and syntocinon 5 units) is given intramuscularly as the anterior shoulder delivers. The oxytocic injection causes the uterus to contract strongly and the placenta to separate almost at once. Having ascertained that the uterus is contracted, the left hand is placed on the abdomen above the symphysis holding the contracted uterus out of the pelvis. The right hand exerts steady firm downward pressure on the cord. The active management of the third stage has reduced the overall blood loss at delivery and the number of cases of haemorrhage. The placenta and membranes must be carefully examined for completeness, and the cord inspected to record the number of arteries. If one of the two arteries is absent, fetal abnormalities may be present.

The mother must not be left alone for at least an hour after delivery, and during this time the uterus must be frequently palpated and blood loss observed to detect any bleeding. The pulse and blood pressure are recorded. Any episiotomy or lacerations are sutured as soon after delivery as possible with further careful infiltration of additional local anaesthetic.

The baby should be put to the breast at the earliest moment before weighing, measuring and attending to the cord, all of which removes the baby from the mother. The mother and father should be offered the traditional cup of tea and then, with the mother in a comfortable bed, her baby in a cot beside her, with a firmly contracted uterus and no bleeding, she is encouraged to sleep.

Episiotomy

This is an incision made with scissors in the perineum after infiltration with local anaesthetic (e.g. 10 ml of 0·5 per cent lignocaine) along the line of the incision. Incision starts in the midline and is carried in a postero-lateral direction to avoid the anal sphincter. (See Fig. 14.4.) The exact line of the episiotomy may be dictated by vulval varices, which should be avoided, or previous episiotomy scars, which should be refashioned.

Indications

1. Prevent incipient tearing of the perineum.
2. Remove obstruction during delivery of the head of the premature infant and thus prevent rapid changes in intracranial pressure.
3. Facilitate intravaginal manoeuvres, i.e. the application of forceps, and give protection to maternal tissues.

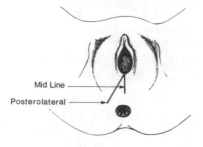

Fig. 14.4. Episiotomy.

Complications

1. The episiotomy may extend if it is too small or care is not taken at delivery, particularly of the posterior shoulder. The tear usually turns medially, tracking down towards the anal margin, and may involve the sphincter and even rectum. The vaginal part of the episiotomy may tear up the posterolateral vaginal wall.
2. Bleeding may be profuse, particularly if an intravaginal tear is not recognized.
3. Other complications are dealt with under Maternal Trauma, later in this chapter.

INDUCTION OF LABOUR

Those attendant upon pregnant women throughout the ages have tried to induce labour for various reasons in various ways, from herbal potions to Indian braves on horseback leaping across the prostrate patient. For centuries before the advent of antibiotics, the risks of infection with its dire consequences to both mother and baby if the membranes were ruptured were recognized. Artificial rupture of the membranes is now the common way of inducing labour, but this procedure should never be undertaken lightly because failure leads to Caesarean section and still occasionally to sepsis. It is to be regarded as a surgical procedure and therefore scrupulous attention must be paid to asepsis. It should only be carried out in a maternity unit fully equipped to proceed to Caesarean section at a moment's notice.

The indications for induction of labour are numerous and are discussed in the relevant sections in the previous chapter. Briefly reviewed they are:

pre-eclampsia/hypertension;
postmaturity;
antepartum bleeding;
placental insufficiency;
diabetes;
rhesus haemolytic disease;

fetal abnormality or death;

multiple pregnancy.

The prerequisites for induction are a longitudinal fetal lie and a presenting part in the pelvis. A favourable cervix (that is soft, effaced and 2 cm dilated) is not an absolute prerequisite but the state of the cervix is a guide to how readily the patient will go into labour after induction. The Bishop's score is a way of expressing the factors relating to ease of induction and is used in many units.

Bishop's score = inducibility rating

	0 cm	1–2 cm	3–4 cm	5–6 cm
Dilatation of cervix	0 cm	1–2 cm	3–4 cm	5–6 cm
Score	0	1	2	3
Effacement	0–30%	40–50%	60–70%	80–100%
Score	0	1	2	3
Station of presenting part	−3 cm	−2 cm	−1, 0 cm	+1, +2 cm
Score	0	1	2	3
Consistency of cervix	Firm	Medium	Soft	
Score	0	1	2	
Position of cervix	Posterior	Mid position	Anterior	
Score	0	1	2	

Total Score   0– 5 = Unfavourable
                  6–13 = Favourable

Dangers of Induction

The dangers of induction are:

1. failure to establish labour;
2. sepsis, fetal and maternal;
3. prolapse of the cord;
4. wrong dates – prematurity.

Although induction of labour is usually successful, should labour fail to become established and the patient seem unlikely to deliver with 24 hours she will require a Caesarean section. Infection of the membranes (chorionitis or amnionitis), intrapartum fetal pneumonia and endometritis are all sequelae of prolonged rupture of the membranes (more than 24 hours), but infective complications have been recorded after much shorter times. If the presenting part is not in the pelvis the cord may prolapse. Any uncertainty about maturity may result in the delivery of a premature infant.

Methods of Induction

Amniotomy
    low (forewaters)
    high (historical only)

Oxytocic agents
intravenously
orally (sublingual)
extra/intra-amniotically.

The usual method of induction is by artificial rupture of the membranes (ARM). The membranes ruptured are those below the presenting part, i.e. the forewaters (low amniotomy).

Procedure for Induction of Labour

1. Review the indications.
2. Reassess maturity.

(An enema is only needed if the patient is constipated. Her pubic hair only needs shaving if it is particularly profuse.)

3. Abdominal palpation confirms the fetal lie (which must be longitudinal) and the position of the presenting part which should be in the pelvis (at least partly). The fetal heart is auscultated.
4. The patient is placed in lithotomy position and a vaginal examination is carried out to check pelvic capacity, the position and station of the presenting part and the state of the cervix. If there is no suspicion of placenta praevia one or two fingers are passed through the cervix and the membranes are swept off the lower segment and the cervix is stretched. This procedure alone often stimulates contractions, probably due to a release of prostaglandins. The forewaters are ruptured with an amniotomy hook, Kocher's forceps or a similar instrument.
5. The colour and amount of liquor are noted. If bleeding occurs, the blood should be analysed at once for fetal haemoglobin. Undetected rupture of vasa praevia may result in an exsanguinated fetus.
6. After ARM prolapse of the cord should be excluded by vaginal examination.
7. Dictated to some extent by the Bishop's score, an intravenous infusion of syntocinon may be set up at the same time as ARM if the score is unfavourable or after a few hours if contractions have not started, even with a favourable score.

Rupture of the hindwaters (high amniotomy) with the sigmoid-shaped Drew Smythe catheter has no place now since there is increased risk of placental damage with this procedure, the induction delivery interval is longer and the forewaters are often inadvertently ruptured in any case. Sublingual tablets of oxytocin and prostaglandin may be used but absorption is variable and they are not widely used except for the initial ripening of an unfavourable cervix. Tetanic uterine contraction has occurred as a complication of oxytocics given by this route. Prostaglandins may be given as vaginal pessaries to ripen the cervix and produce a more favourable Bishop's score. They may also be given intra- or extra-amniotically and are especially useful in cases of fetal abnormality or death. Intra-amniotic prostaglandins usually cause fetal death. Prostaglandins are appreciably more effective than oxytocin in the mid-trimester or with an unfavourable cervix at other times.

Dangers of Intravenous Syntocinon
1. Hypertonic uterine contractions.
2. Spasm.
3. Uterine rupture.
4. Fetal hypoxia.

All of these complications are extremely rare if the course of labour is carefully monitored.

Abnormal Labour (Dystocia)

Abnormal labour may be due to maternal or fetal faults or a combination.

Maternal faults may be due to abnormal uterine activity (hypercontractility, hypocontractility or constriction ring) or to abnormal passages (cervical dystocia, vaginal septa or pelvic tumours).

Fetomaternal faults are due to disproportion (cephalopelvic).

Fetal faults may be due to malposition (OP, face, brow), malpresentation (breech, shoulder, cord) or to abnormality (e.g. hydrocephaly).

Abnormal Uterine Activity

Hypertonic uterine action. Here the contractions are too frequent and there is a high resting tone in the uterus and the contractions are painful. This situation causes maternal exhaustion, and the likelihood of fetal hypoxia is high. Although analgesics such as morphine and pethidine may reduce the contractions these drugs cross the placenta depressing the fetal respiratory centre. An epidural anaesthetic also reduces the strength of the contractions but without affecting the fetus. Caesarean section is sometimes necessary if fetal distress or maternal exhaustion develops. It is essential to monitor the strength of uterine contractions when a syntocinon infusion is used because of the risk of hyperstimulation and tetanic contractions leading to fetal hypoxia.

Hypotonic uterine action. Here the contractions are irregular and infrequent. They are also ineffectual. Adequate uterine action is achieved with intravenous syntocinon and rupture of the membranes. Hypotonic uterine action developing late in labour is nearly always secondary to dehydration and ketosis.

Constriction ring. This is very rare and may follow administration of an oxytocic. It is a localized, persistent area of spasm around the uterus and may occur around the neck of the fetus or cause the placenta to be retained after delivery.

Abnormal Passages

Cervical dystocia. This condition is also rare. Usually failure of cervical dilatation is due to inadequate uterine activity, but occasionally following cervical cautery or cone biopsy the cervix may fail to dilate. Very rarely there is no history of cervical cautery or trauma.

A *vaginal septum* may prevent descent of the head but this is a most unusual occurrence.

Rarely, *tumours* such as a cervical fibromyoma or an ovarian cyst may cause obstructed labour by occupying part of the pelvis.

Malposition

Malposition of the fetal head is when some part of the fetal head other than the vertex presents, for example occipitoposterior or occipitolateral presentation. A malpresentation is when some part of the fetus other than the head presents.

Occipitoposterior Position

The commonest malposition is the occipitoposterior position (OP). This is the usual cause of a high head at term in the primigravida. The head is incompletely flexed and a larger than usual diameter, the occipitofrontal diameter, presents. At the onset of labour the head usually flexes and the malposition is corrected. The occiput may remain posterior after the onset of labour in about 20 per cent of cases.

CAUSES OF OP POSITION
1. Android-shaped pelvis.
2. Anthropoid-shaped pelvis.
3. Epidural analgesia.

DIAGNOSIS OF OP

Abdominal palpation reveals fetal limbs over the front of the uterus. The back is not felt in the flank and there is flattening of the abdomen below the umbilicus. On vaginal examination the anterior fontanelle is readily palpable anteriorly and the posterior fontanelle may be palpated in the posterior part of the pelvis.

MECHANISM OF LABOUR WITH OP

The occiput is frequently posterior at the onset of labour, but the uterine contractions cause flexion of the fetal head, which enters the pelvic brim with the sagittal suture in the transverse diameter. Contractions cause further flexion, which brings the occiput below the sinciput making it the lowest part of the head, and it thus reaches the pelvic floor and rotates anteriorly.

If the contractions fail to bring about adequate flexion the head will enter the brim with the occiput in the posterior position, usually not a direct occipitoposterior position but with the occiput lying in the right oblique diameter of the pelvis, i.e. a right occipitoposterior position (an ROP). As this means that a bigger presenting diameter is coming into the pelvis it may take longer for the head to get into the pelvis; also this less flexed head is a poor fit against the lower segment and therefore not such a good stimulator of contractions. It may be necessary for quite considerable moulding of the fetal head to take place for the head to be able to enter the pelvis and very frequently caput forms. If the pelvis is big enough and in the presence of good uterine contractions, the head may reach the pelvic floor and the occiput may rotate the long way round the pelvis to an occipito-anterior position and the baby deliver by the normal mechanism. If the pelvis is roomy the head may rotate to a direct occipitoposterior position and deliver as a persistent occipitoposterior (POP) with the baby's face delivering beneath the symphysis pubis (face to pubis).

MANAGEMENT OF LABOUR WITH OP
In either of these instances it can be seen that a longer than normal labour is anticipated and it is therefore important to maintain the patient's morale and ensure that she does not become dehydrated. Adequate analgesia is also necessary. In spite of the risk of producing poor levator tone and possible problems with rotation of the fetal head, epidural analgesia is especially helpful to patients with an occipitoposterior position. It is essential to ensure adequate uterine contractions and intravenous syntocinon is usually required, especially after epidural analgesia. Careful monitoring of the fetal heart rate and regular inspection of the liquor is necessary as labour may be prolonged.

If spontaneous delivery does not occur the situation must be assessed carefully. If after phase 1 of the second stage, when the vagina has dilated and the head has reached the perineum, the head has failed to rotate in spite of adequate contractions and an adequate outlet, it will have to be rotated to an occipito-anterior position in order that delivery may occur. Manual rotation of the head may be followed by spontaneous delivery if the mother is not too exhausted but is more usually completed with obstetric forceps. Manual rotation is safe for both mother and baby. Rotation of the head with Kjelland's forceps or the ventouse is not advocated in the authors' unit because of fetal and maternal trauma, but is practised in many hospitals (see under Forceps Delivery in this chapter p. 235). The risks of postpartum haemorrhage are increased since labour may have been prolonged and an operative delivery has occurred. Because of these factors there is an increased perinatal mortality and morbidity due to hypoxia, and birth trauma if forceps have been used. The latter is greatly reduced if manual rotation is employed.

One of the commonest mistakes in obstetrics is to assume that because the cervix is fully dilated the baby is ready to and can be delivered vaginally. Never is this truer than in the case of occipitoposterior presentation where caput and moulding may appear at the vulva, leading the unwary obstetrician to assume all is ready for forceps delivery. In reality the head is above the pelvic floor, often still palpable abdominally and the patient should be delivered by Caesarean section. Forceps delivery should not be undertaken unless the vagina is dilated and the head is on the pelvic floor, phase 1 of the second stage having been completed. This is true for occipito-anterior and occipitoposterior positions. Misdiagnosis or misguided attempts at delivery with either presentation, but particularly with the occipitoposterior. lead to a greatly increased perinatal mortality and morbidity and severe maternal trauma in many cases.

Deep Transverse Arrest
This is a separate entity. Here the head has entered the pelvic brim with the sagittal suture in the transverse diameter of the brim, but as the contractions cause less flexion than usual the occiput and sinciput remain at the same level. The head remains in this position as it descends through the pelvis and fails to rotate either anteriorly or posteriorly becoming arrested in the transverse position. When a deep transverse arrest is diagnosed its cause must be sought. Are uterine contractions adequate to help the head to flex? Is there reasonable tone in the pelvic floor? Is the pelvis a normal shape? The criteria for delivery of the deep transverse arrest are exactly those for the occipitoposterior position. If the head reaches the perineum in the second phase of the second stage then rotation may easily be effected manually and the head delivered with the occiput anterior with little risk to mother or baby. If the head remains in the transverse position at the level of the ischial spines in spite of full dilatation of cervix, then operative delivery is likely to be hazardous for fetus and mother, and abdominal delivery should be undertaken.

Face Presentation
The incidence of face presentation is 1 in 300. The commonest cause is anencephaly, i.e. there is no cranium to the fetal head. Hypertonus in the extensor muscles of the fetal neck is said to be a cause of face presentation and the baby delivered as a face often lies in its cot with its neck extended for several days after birth. The cause of the hypertonus is unknown. Rarely a thyroid tumour or hypoglossal cyst may cause the head to be extended. A lax uterus or hydramnios may predispose to extension of the head and face presentation.

DIAGNOSIS OF FACE PRESENTATION
This is rarely made before labour but if it is, concern about fetal abnormality is aroused. On abdominal examination the hyperextended chest feels like the normal fetal back but lies on the same side as the feet. On vaginal examination oedema always makes palpation of soft fetal parts difficult, but the supraorbital ridges and bridge of the nose are felt. A face

presentation is not uncommonly misdiagnosed as a breech. An X-ray confirms the diagnosis and excludes anencephaly as a cause.

MANAGEMENT OF FACE PRESENTATION

When the head is fully extended and the face presents, the presenting diameter is the submentobregmatic (9·5 cm), the same as the suboccipito-bregmatic which presents with the fully flexed head. The head engages in the transverse diameter of the pelvis, the chin (mentum) being used as the denominator rather than the occiput. As descent occurs the chin reaches the pelvic floor and usually rotates anteriorly coming under the pubis, and delivery of the head is by flexion. If the chin rotates posteriorly (a mento-posterior position) further descent and delivery could only occur if the neck extended further, and delivery must be by Caesarean section as the head and neck are already fully extended.

OUTCOME

Since the malposition is often associated with fetal abnormality there is a high overall fetal mortality. Since operative delivery is frequently necessary, maternal and fetal morbidity is increased.

Brow Presentation

Here the head is midway between extension and flexion. The largest diameter of the skull, the mentovertical, is the presenting diameter. Since this in the normal-size term infant (i.e. 3·5 kg) measures 13·5 cm it is apparent that delivery is impossible. The incidence of a brow presentation is 1 : 1000 and its cause is unknown.

DIAGNOSIS OF BROW

On abdominal palpation the head feels big and is not engaged. On vaginal examination the anterior fontanelle is presenting and the supraorbital ridges can be felt. An X-ray confirms the diagnosis and is often requested to exclude hydrocephaly since this is the impression obtained on abdominal palpation. Since the presenting part does not fit the lower segment the membranes may rupture early and the cord prolapse.

MANAGEMENT

In early labour it is reasonable to wait a few hours to see whether with adequate uterine contractions the brow converts to a face by increasing extension, or an occipito-anterior position by increasing flexion, but this expectant attitude cannot be maintained for long otherwise labour will become obstructed. If the brow persists then delivery is by Caesarean section.

OUTCOME

Operative delivery will increase the maternal morbidity, but fetal mortality and morbidity should be low if Caesarean section is carried out early.

Malpresentation

The commonest malpresentation is the breech and is discussed in Chapter 13. It is emphasized again here that the decision to allow the patient with a breech presentation to go into labour and attempt a vaginal delivery is only taken after very careful antenatal assessment together with constant assessment as to the progress of labour, particularly the rapidity of the descent of the breech. The patient having a baby by the breech must be delivered in a major obstetric unit, supervised by a senior experienced obstetrician and be attended by an anaesthetist and a paediatrician. If, in spite of full dilatation, the breech has not reached the perineum, the fetus should be delivered by Caesarean section.

Management of Breech Delivery

With the breech distending the perineum the patient is asked to bear down with contractions. In order to aid delivery of the baby the patient is in lithotomy position. She is swabbed and draped and her bladder emptied. At full distension of the perineum an episiotomy is made to be used later to assist delivery of the head. The patient continues to bear down with contractions. If the legs do not deliver spontaneously gentle pressure behind the knee joints causing the leg to flex will enable the foot to be flipped over the perineum. It is essential to keep the fetal back uppermost and a towel may be wrapped around the fetal pelvis and the operator may hold the fetal pelvis with his thumbs lying along the back of the sacrum. He must not grasp the baby around its abdominal cavity as this can cause trauma to the intra-abdominal organs, particularly the liver. It is important that no traction at all is applied to the fetus. The purpose of holding the fetus is to maintain the back anteriorly. The mother continues to bear down as the shoulders come into view. The arms may deliver spontaneously; if not, gentle pressure in the antecubital fossa to cause the arm to flex will allow the arm to be flipped out. The Løvset manoeuvre is useful for delivering extended arms, but extended arms rarely arise spontaneously and are usually produced as the result of injudicious traction on the fetus. The Løvset manoeuvre involves rotating the fetus through 180° to bring the erstwhile posterior shoulder anteriorly to lie directly under the symphysis pubis so that the arm may be brought down across the face and delivered; rotation in the opposite direction allows delivery of the other arm.

Gravity and the mother's expulsive efforts should bring the head into the pelvis with the next contraction and the occiput will appear below the symphysis. When this is seen the feet are held gently in the left hand and raised vertically and then held by an assistant. The head is delivered by forceps in a slow controlled manner to avoid damage.

Breech delivery should not be hurried, but it is obvious that it should not be too prolonged either since the baby's oxygen supply via the placenta is increasingly reduced as delivery proceeds, and the baby is not able to take a breath until the head has been delivered. Delivery of a baby by the breech should take no more than 5–8 minutes at the very most.

Variable Lie and Shoulder Presentation

During the latter weeks of pregnancy the fetal lie usually stabilizes with the breech or head presenting, the lie being longitudinal. In highly parous patients with lax anterior abdominal walls, patients with gross spinal curvature and a pendulous abdomen and occasionally patients with a space-occupying lesion of the lower segment or pelvis (e.g. placenta praevia or fibroids) the lie may be variable or persistently transverse. This may occur in the primigravida too but less commonly. Often no obvious cause is found for the abnormal lie.

During pregnancy, management is expectant since the lie usually becomes longitudinal spontaneously by 38 weeks. If it does not the patient is admitted to hospital at that time, since should the membranes rupture there is a very real danger that the cord may prolapse, and should contractions occur and the lie remain transverse the shoulder will impact in the pelvis. The arm may prolapse and labour will become obstructed. Before 38 weeks the patient is urged to report immediately should she suspect that her membranes have ruptured or that labour may have started. Expectant treatment continues in hospital. If the membranes rupture and the cord prolapses, immediate Caesarean section should be carried out. If labour starts with a transverse or varying lie, Caesarean section should be undertaken. In the majority of cases, however, the lie stabilizes spontaneously by 41 weeks and labour starts with a longitudinal lie. If the lie remains variable or transverse approaching 42 weeks, elective Caesarean section is arranged, after confirming the maturity of the fetus. External cephalic version is usually a waste of time at any period of gestation since the abnormal lie recurs; once contractions have started it is very difficult, and if the membranes have ruptured it is impossible.

MULTIPLE PREGNANCY

Since twins are the commonest multiple they will be considered in detail. Triplets may be delivered vaginally but Caesarean section is often done for multiples greater than 2.

Diagnosed Twins

During labour it is necessary to monitor the heart of both infants. A scalp clip may be applied to the presenting part of twin 1, and twin 2 may be monitored externally. It is important to anticipate the problems attendant on twin delivery.

Problems

The problems which may arise with twin 2 in the second stage are:
    abnormal lie;

abnormal presentation;

intrauterine anoxia.

The problems associated with the third stage are:

postpartum haemorrhage;

uterine atony.

An intravenous infusion must be running before the second stage begins. The following personnel should be in attendance when the second stage begins:

1. An experienced obstetrician who can carry out intrauterine manipulations and a Caesarean section.
2. An anaesthetist.
3. At least one paediatrician and preferably two, as twins are often premature and may be small.

Twin 1

The delivery of the first twin is managed as it would be for a singleton with the same presentation. The cord must be cut between two clamps as usual. This is particularly important as bleeding from the cut end of the cord leading to the placenta may cause exsanguination of twin 2 if there is an anastomotic connection between the fetal circulations in the placentae.

Twin 2

As soon as twin 1 has delivered, abdominal palpation should be carried out to ascertain the lie and presentation of twin 2, and its heart auscultated. External manipulation will usually correct an oblique or transverse lie. The membranes are ruptured with the next contraction and certainly within 5 minutes of the delivery of twin 1. The obstetrician's hand is kept in the vagina after rupture of the membranes to exclude cord prolapse and to guide the presenting part. The patient is encouraged to bear down. Contractions may be stimulated with syntocinon if they are slow to re-establish. The second twin is at ever-increasing risk from hypoxia and placental separation once twin 1 has delivered and the size of the uterus decreases. If there is any delay in descent then forceps may be applied to the head or the breech extracted by gentle traction on the legs.

A manoeuvre is permissible in relation to twin delivery that has no other place in modern obstetric practice – this is internal version and breech extraction. If the head is presenting and remains high above the pelvic brim, or if the lie is transverse or the cord prolapses, then a hand can be introduced into the uterus, the fetal foot sought, being recognized by the calcaneum, and the leg brought down. The baby is then extracted by pulling on the leg which straightens out the lie and brings the breech down into the pelvis. This manoeuvre can only be done with any degree of safety to mother and baby in the case of twin 2, where the birth canal has been dilated by twin 1 and the membranes of the second sac only just ruptured. Uterine rupture and fetal death are the ultimate hazards of this manoeuvre.

Undiagnosed Twins

If a second fetus is suspected before the second stage is complete no oxytocic is given. However, the more common situation is that the second twin is found after the delivery of the first and after the oxytocic has been given. The abdomen should be palpated and the fetal lie made longitudinal; the membranes ruptured and twin 2 delivered as expeditiously as possible with internal version and breech extraction if necessary.

OBSTETRICAL MANOEUVRES

Amniocentesis (see Chapter 13).
Induction of labour (see p. 224).
Episiotomy (see p. 223).

Pudendal Block

Blocking the pudendal nerve provides adequate perineal analgesia for mid- and low-cavity pelvic manipulations.

The pudendal nerve curves around the ischial spine and supplies the skin of the vulva. Infiltration of 10 ml of lignocaine 1 per cent just beneath the ischial spine will produce introital analgesia. The infiltration may be made transvaginally or percutaneously using a long 10 cm needle. With the latter route a bleb of local anaesthetic is injected intradermally midway between the anus and the ischial tuberosity. The needle is passed through the bleb and directed to the ischial spine. With both routes a finger in the vagina directs the needle towards the ischial spine. It is necessary to infiltrate the perineum posteriorly, especially along the line of a proposed episiotomy.

Forceps Delivery

Obstetrical forceps were invented in the seventeenth century by the Chamberlen family and kept in secret use by members of the family for over 100 years. The instruments were covered in leather to prevent them making a noise and giving a clue about the Chamberlen's secret instrument.

There are two main types of modern forceps: those for applying traction and those for rotating and applying traction.

Simple Traction Forceps

1. Long curved forceps (e.g. Neville Barnes) are for mid-cavity deliveries.
2. Short curved forceps (e.g. Wrigleys) are for low 'lift out' deliveries where the head is on the perineum.

There is no place for high forceps delivery where the head is above the pelvic brim. The risk of trauma to mother and fetus is too great. Mid-cavity deliveries should be undertaken only after very careful assessment, as in many cases vaginal dilatation has not taken place and the head is still above the pelvic floor. The forceps consist of two parts, each part having a blade and a handle. The blade is curved to fit the fetal head and also to fit the pelvis. Each blade is applied separately (the left always first), care being taken that the blade is correctly positioned along the side of the fetal head. The handle is locked after correct application. The sagittal suture must be in the AP diameter of the pelvis.

Rotational Forceps

Kjelland's forceps. These forceps have a much flatter pelvic curve and are used for rotating the head from occipitoposterior or occipitotransverse positions to occipito-anterior positions. It is a dangerous instrument and rarely used in the authors' obstetric practice, except by senior obstetricians. Rotation of these malpositions can also be accomplished by manual rotation with subsequent extraction using conventional forceps. The dangers to mother and baby have been emphasized above, and the use of Kjelland's forceps is consequently in decline.

Prerequisites for Forceps Delivery

1. The cervix must be fully dilated.
2. There must be no disproportion.
3. The head must be engaged.
4. The occiput must be anterior.
5. The bladder should be empty.
6. The uterus must be contracting.
7. The membranes must be ruptured.

Ideally the vagina should be dilated and the head on the pelvic floor. A lip of cervix may be pushed up at the time of forceps delivery, but special care must be taken if the cervix is not fully dilated, and the indications for forceps delivery must be reassessed by an experienced obstetrician. Forceps delivery in such cases should rarely if ever be contemplated. The cervix may inadvertently be damaged and should always be inspected after forceps delivery. If the head is on the perineum and the occiput remains posterior at the outlet then it is possible to deliver the fetus face to pubis, but in the mid-cavity the occiput should be anterior before attempting forceps delivery. If the uterus is not contracting, postpartum haemorrhage is more likely.

Indications for Forceps Delivery

1. Delay in the second stage. This may be due to ineffectual uterine contractions or poor maternal expulsive efforts. A rigid perineum may also cause delay. Fetal causes of delay include malposition of the fetal head, especially occipitoposterior or occipitotransverse positions. Cephalopelvic disproportion may also cause delay and should be excluded before undertaking forceps delivery. Delay due to ineffectual uterine action may be overcome using syntocinon, and an episiotomy will relieve delay due to a rigid perineum.
2. Maternal distress or exhaustion at this stage is to be regarded as a failure of management, but occasionally the mother is in such a distressed state that she is unable to cooperate and push adequately.

3. Forceps delivery is also indicated when a short second stage is necessary (e.g. cardiac patients, those with severe hypertension or those who have had a previous Caesarean section). It is important that the patient who is delivering a baby prematurely should also have a short second stage, and delivery of the head should be controlled as precipitate delivery (particularly of the premature head) may cause tentorial tears with subsequent damage or death. Forceps may be applied to the head of the premature infant to control its delivery, but it must be remembered that the premature head is more vulnerable that at term and the forceps themselves may cause damage. An adequate episiotomy will facilitate the delivery of the premature head more safely than forceps.

Fetal distress may occur for the first time in the second stage and is usually due to hypoxia. It should be watched for carefully, especially if there is an underlying cause for fetal distress such as placental insufficiency.

Dangers of Forceps Delivery

Injudicious or unskilled use of any type of forceps may damage mother or fetus. Vaginal and cervical lacerations, uterine rupture, vesicovaginal fistulae, rectovaginal fistulae and postpartum haemorrhage may all follow forceps delivery. Fetal death may occur from intracranial haemorrhage and the fetal skull may be fractured. Facial palsy results from inaccurate application of the blades. Cerebral irritation is frequently seen, particularly after rotational forceps delivery, and cerebral damage resulting in long-term morbidity is sadly not uncommon. The use of forceps is under review and likely to decrease.

Ventouse

This instrument consists of a metal cup and chain which is attached to a vacuum bottle. The cup (which comes in 3 sizes) is placed on the fetal scalp and a negative pressure of 9·8 kg per cm^2 is established in not less than 8 minutes which sucks the scalp into the cup, forming a chignon. Traction may then be applied.

The ventouse may be used in place of forceps and in certain developing countries is widely used by semi-skilled childbirth attendants since less expertise is needed. In cases of fetal distress it is slower to use than forceps. Scalp damage may be caused if application is prolonged. It is possible, but inadvisable, to apply the ventouse before the cervix is fully dilated where there is delay in the first stage, as maternal and fetal damage may follow. Since disproportion is a common cause for such delay, ventouse extraction is to be avoided, since gross fetal and maternal damage may result. The ventouse has no place in the authors' obstetric practice.

Caesarean Section .

Julius Caesar was not delivered by this operation, in spite of the name. Under Roman law the fetus had to be taken from the body of a mother dying during pregnancy or labour and the operation thus became known as Caesarean section. It was not until the late nineteenth century that the classical section was perfected and only in the early twentieth century that the lower segment operation was devised. Caesarean section did not become safe until the advent of blood transfusion and antibiotics, and even today is occasionally a direct cause of maternal death.

Indications

Caesarean section is undertaken for a variety of indications, mentioned in Chapter 13. Briefly reviewed they are:

Fetal Indications

Fetal distress in first stage.
Inadequate placental reserve, e.g. growth retardation.
Diabetes.

Maternal Indications

Previous Caesarean section for recurrent cause.
Two or more previous Caesarean sections.
Some previous gynaecological surgery, e.g. repair of fistula, repair of prolapse.

Combined Indications

Antepartum haemorrhage.
Cephalopelvic disproportion.
Malpresentation.
Malposition.
Hypertensive disorders.

Method

If Caesarean section is the elective method of delivery then it is done about a week before term. More usually it is done as an emergency procedure in labour. Since particularly in labour there is delayed gastric emptying, with the hazards of aspiration of acid gastric contents, and the possibility of anaesthesia is always present, patients in labour are not fed but are given an antacid every 2 hours.

General anaesthesia is commonly used, but epidural anaesthesia is gaining popularity and has the advantage that the mother may see and hold her baby almost immediately. A skilled obstetric anaesthetist should be available and 2 units of blood should be cross matched.

Fig. 14.5 indicates the merits of the lower segment incision and the problems associated with the classical section.

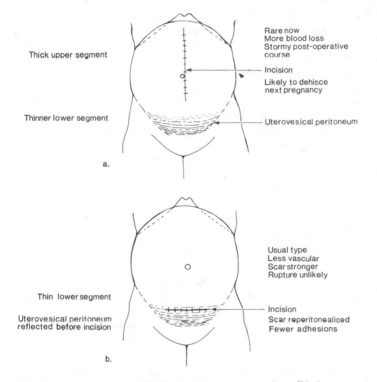

Fig. 14.5. Caesarean section. (a) Classical Caesarean section. (b) Lower segment Caesarean section.

Postpartum Haemorrhage

Primary postpartum haemorrhage is defined as a loss of 500 ml or more within the first 24 hours after birth. The incidence is approximately 1 to 2 per cent.

Causes of Postpartum Haemorrhage

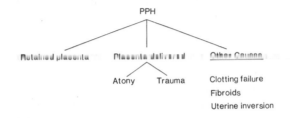

Fig. 14.6.

Retained Placenta

Partial separation of the placenta interferes with uterine contraction, and the maternal sinuses of the separated part of the placenta are held open and bleed. If the placenta fails to separate at all, as in the very rare cases of morbid adherence (e.g. placenta accreta), there is no bleeding since the sinuses are not exposed. It is more usual for some separation to occur followed by haemorrhage. If the placenta separates completely but is retained in the lower segment due to contraction of the cervix, this too will interfere with contraction of the fundus and placental site and pre-dispose to haemorrhage.

Uterine Atony

If the uterus has been overdistended (for example in polyhydramnios, multiple pregnancy or with a large baby) it may fail to contract after delivery. Atony is more common after a long exhausting labour and if deep anaesthesia is used.

Lacerations

Tears anywhere in the genital tract from vulva and vagina through the cervix to the uterus that are unrecognized or inadequately repaired may cause bleeding. Operative vaginal delivery or intrauterine manipulations will increase the likelihood of trauma to the genital tract.

Other Causes

Clotting defects rarely cause postpartum haemorrhage because haemostasis relies primarily on uterine muscle contraction and retraction. Clotting failure may cause serious problems if associated with inefficient uterine action, and may happen, for instance, with a severe abruptio placentae. Uterine fibroids may interfere with efficient contraction of the uterus and predispose to haemorrhage. Injudicious traction on the cord of the un-separated placenta may cause uterine inversion, although occasionally inversion occurs spontaneously.

Diagnosis of Postpartum Haemorrhage

All blood loss at delivery is measured, but it is notoriously difficult for the collection to be complete. It has also been shown that estimates of blood loss are usually completely erroneous, the assessment made being far too little. The larger the volume lost the more inaccurate is the assessment.

Management of Postpartum Haemorrhage

1. Stop the bleeding.
2. Resuscitate the patient.

The first step is to give ergometrine 0·5 mg intravenously. The second is to rub up a uterine contraction. Ten ml of blood for cross matching are taken and an intravenous infusion is set up. If there are enough personnel these steps can be in progress while the cause of the postpartum haemorrhage is being sought. If the placenta is retained it must be removed. If the placenta is delivered it must be examined for completeness. In either event, if the uterus is atonic and full of blood clot a contraction must be rubbed up and the clots expelled. If the uterus fails to remain contracted a continuous intravenous infusion of syntocinon is set up (20 units of syntocinon in 500 ml of dextrose saline). Bimanual compression of the uterus is very effective and may be life-saving in situations where oxytocics and blood are not available. It is effective as long as the placenta is out. A clenched hand is inserted into the vagina as high as possible and the uterus is compressed on to the vaginal fist by placing the other hand suprapubically on the patient's abdomen holding the fundus down and continuing to rub up a contraction. If uterine bleeding due to atony continues to be a problem, internal iliac artery ligation or hysterectomy may be necessary. There is no place for hot douches or uterine packs. These are a waste of time, predispose to infection and may damage the uterus.

Removal of the Retained Placenta

Even if bleeding is not a feature it may occur at any time and therefore an intravenous infusion should be set up and blood cross matched. Manual removal should be carried out under general anaesthesia, since to put a hand into the uterus may provoke shock.

Before anaesthesia is induced, controlled cord traction is performed after ensuring the uterus is contracted, since separation may have occurred in the meanwhile.

After anaesthesia is induced, the patient's bladder must be emptied and a hand slipped through the cerivx following the cord up to the placenta. The edge of the placenta is sought. The uterus is steadied by the operator's other hand which is holding the uterus through the anterior abdominal wall. The placenta is lifted off the uterine wall, not clawed off in pieces. The uterine cavity is then re-explored to remove any fragments left behind. Ergometrine 0·5 mg is given intravenously at the end of the procedure.

Manual removal of the placenta should only be undertaken by an experienced obstetrician, with the strictest aseptic precautions, with expert anaesthesia and with blood available.

Should a patient deliver away from a major unit and the placenta be retained, then the obstetric flying squad should be called. The placenta should be removed before any attempt is made to transfer the patient.

The first *Report on Confidential Enquiries into Maternal Deaths in England and Wales 1952–1954* (see Chapter 16) showed that transfer of a patient with the placenta in situ was a major cause of death, the patient not infrequently bleeding during transfer and arriving dead or moribund at the major unit.

Lacerations

If bleeding continues after delivery in spite of a well-contracted uterus the genital tract must be inspected. This should be carried out with the patient in lithotomy position under general anaesthesia with operating theatre facilities.

The episiotomy or tear may not be adequately sutured at the top end. It may have extended into the posterior fornix.

A vaginal haematoma may be accumulating from an undetected vaginal wall laceration.

The cervix may be torn, especially at 3 and 9 o'clock. The apex of any tear must be defined to ensure that the tear does not extend into the uterus.

The uterine cavity must be gently explored to confirm its integrity.

Clotting Defects

These are usually suspected either following a history of abruption or when it is noticed that the blood taken for cross matching does not clot, the patient is oozing from the site of venepuncture and the blood from the genital tract fails to clot.

The common defect is hypofibrinogenaemia, and the fibrinogen level and fibrinogen degradation products may be measured to confirm the diagnosis. Treatment is most effective when absolutely fresh blood is transfused. However, fibrinogen may be given.

Sequelae of Primary PPH

Five per cent of maternal deaths are due to postpartum haemorrhage and over half of these are avoidable. Following hypovolaemic shock there is renal shutdown, anuria and possibly irreparable renal damage. Chronic anaemia in the puerperium, which is responsible for many minor ills, irritability, tiredness, depression, apathy, insomnia and so on, often goes unrecognized and frequently follows the less dramatic postpartum haemorrhage.

Prolonged hypotension may cause damage to the blood supply to the pituitary resulting in panhypopituitarism (Sheehan's syndrome). The features are not usually apparent until several weeks or months after delivery, but it should be suspected if lactation fails to become established.

Secondary PPH

This is discussed in Chapter 15.

Maternal Trauma

The Vulva

A vulval haematoma is readily diagnosed. The very painful tense collection of blood is due to rupture of a subcutaneous blood vessel. The haematoma must be incised, the clot evacuated and the bleeding vessel ligated if it can be found.

The Perineum

First degree tear involves the skin only at the fourchette, *2nd degree tear* involves the perineal body and posterior vaginal wall and *3rd degree tear* involves the external anal sphincter and often the anal mucosa as well as the posterior vaginal wall.

All tears need careful repair. Dyspareunia is commonly seen following inadequate or overenthusiastic repair, and in later life prolapse may occur if the perineal body is not reconstituted correctly. An unrecognized or ill-repaired third degree tear leaves the patient incontinent of faeces and flatus.

Repair should be undertaken immediately after delivery since oedema will obscure the field if repair is delayed. The greater the tear the greater the skill required for adequate suture.

Adequate analgesia, exposure, lighting and experience are necessary for satisfactory repair of a tear or episiotomy. The distress caused by improper repair is not seen till much later after discharge and then rarely by the person responsible for the suturing. Vulval and perineal oedema can be very distressing, as can prolapsed haemorrhoids. Ice packs and sitting on a rubber ring or sheepskin will ease the condition locally. Oral analgesics are required.

The Vagina

Lacerations must be defined and repaired. General anaesthesia may be required and certainly adequate exposure, lighting, experience and an assistant are necessary. A vaginal haematoma may occur during delivery, either from spontaneous rupture of a subcutaneous blood vessel or from an undetected laceration. There may be no visible blood loss. The patient usually complains of perineal pain or of a continuing desire to bear down after delivery of the fetus and placenta. Blood transfusion may be needed and the patient should be resuscitated before the haematoma is evacuated. It is rarely possible to see a bleeding point. Sometimes the cavity can be obliterated by mattress sutures, but at other times firm packing is required to obtain haemostasis. Fistulae are rare in the UK, but in some remote areas abroad prolonged obstructed labour not infrequently produces vesicovaginal or rectovaginal fistulae through pressure necrosis. The anterior wall must be inspected for tears after rotational forceps.

The Cervix

Small tears are common and of little importance but larger tears which often occur at 3 and 9 o'clock may extend into the lower uterine segment or into the broad ligament. A broad ligament haematoma may be palpable abdominally and will displace the uterus laterally. Transfusion is usually required but the haematoma will resolve spontaneously. This may take several weeks. Rarely it becomes infected and then has to be drained.

The Uterus
Inversion of the Uterus

Inversion usually occurs when cord traction has been applied before placental separation and in the absence of uterine contractions. It is rare but should be recognized at once since immediate replacement forestalls shock, which may be fatal. The fundus may appear at the introitus or be felt in the vagina, and the uterus will be impalpable on abdominal examination.

Shock occurs because of traction on the tubes and ovaries, which are drawn down into the inverted fundus. Shock may be avoided if immediate replacement is carried out, before the uterus has contracted. If there is delay the inverted fundus becomes fixed in position by the uterus contracting. Bleeding may be profuse. After initial resuscitation, replacement by saline (O'Sullivan's hydrostatic method) is favoured in the UK. The hydrostatic method entails filling the vagina with warm saline while closing the vulva manually to prevent escape. Gradually as the pressure of saline increases the inversion reduces.

Rupture of the Uterus

A complete rupture with tearing of the peritoneal covering may result in extrusion of part or all of the fetus and placenta accompanied by severe haemorrhage. This catastrophic event for both mother and fetus is very rare in the UK today. A rupture occurring in the lower segment may produce a broad ligament haematoma. The rupture may occur at the site of a previous operative scar or in a previously intact uterus.

Scar Rupture

The classical Caesarean section scar ruptures in 3 per cent of cases. Half of these ruptures occur before the onset of labour. Rupture is usually sudden and complete, with death of the fetus and often death of the mother. The lower segment Caesarean section scar ruptures in 0·5 per cent of cases and very rarely occurs before the onset of labour. Rupture is usually gradual and usually diagnosed before the fetus or mother are in serious trouble. Hysterotomy scars carry risks similar to classical Caesarean section scars. Myomectomy scars carry a very small risk of rupture.

Rupture of the previously intact uterus is extremely rare in this country and usually results from some form of obstetric mismanagement such as neglected obstructed labour, particularly in parous women, overdosage of oxytocic drugs, traumatic deliveries or ill-advised intrauterine manoeuvres, such as destructive operations on the fetus other than in very experienced hands. Spontaneous rupture of the previously intact uterus does occur and when it does so it is usually in a grand multipara in labour.

Diagnosis of Uterine Rupture

IN PREGNANCY

The patient may feel the scar 'give way', and this sensation may be associated with pain. If the contents are completely extruded and the uterus contracts there may be little bleeding, shock and pain, but there may be sudden collapse with severe bleeding. The degree of shock and abdominal pain due to intraperitoneal bleeding depends on the amount of bleeding.

IN LABOUR

Rupture of a scar may be silent, and it is not uncommon to find a partial dehiscence at the time of repeat Caesarean section.

Rupture in obstructed labour is usually associated with pain and quite profound shock, since intraperitoneal bleeding is a feature of rupture and the exhausted uterus fails to contract. Infection is usually present too.

IN THE IMMEDIATE PUERPERIUM

If a patient collapses with or without bleeding the possibility of uterine rupture must not be overlooked. The uterus should be explored under general anaesthesia.

Treatment

Resuscitation is the first concern and this includes blood transfusion. If there is doubt about the diagnosis an EUA is done. Having made the diagnosis laparotomy is performed. If the rupture is due to scar dehiscence then simple suture is often all that is required. Hysterectomy is indicated if the uterus is too damaged. If the patient is seen late and in severe shock, haemostatic suturing of the tear should be combined with tubal ligation as hysterectomy carries dangers.

Causes of Shock in Obstetrics

These may be summarized as follows:
    haemorrhage;
    amniotic fluid embolism;
    bacteraemia;
    anoxia and inhalation under anaesthesia;
    pulmonary embolism;
    cardiac failure;
    trauma.

The authors are grateful to Dr Kieran O'Driscoll and Dr Declan Meagher for their advice and recommend their book *Active Management of Labour*, details of which are given below.

Further Reading
O'Driscoll K. and Meagher D. (1980) *Active Management of Labour*. Eastbourne, W. B. Saunders.

Chapter fifteen

Postnatal Care

The puerperium is defined as the time for recovery from the effects of childbearing. The average woman feels fit after 2 weeks, but certain organs take up to 3 months to return to normal.

Physiology and Routine Care

Immediately after delivery the patient is fatigued. The importance of rest is often neglected and adequate sleep should be ensured throughout the puerperium. The temperature at delivery is often subnormal, and shivering is a frequent symptom. In the first 24 hours the temperature rises slightly above normal perhaps as a reaction to catabolism, but should then settle. After this a rise of more than 0·5 °C (1 °F) is abnormal and a cause should be sought.

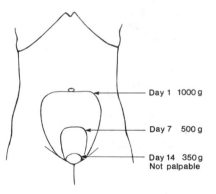

Day 1 1000 g

Day 7   500 g

Day 14 350 g
Not palpable

Fig. 15.1. Involution of the uterus.

Involution of the Genital Tract

Following the abrupt withdrawal of oestrogens as the placenta is delivered, the uterus shrinks by autolysis of the excess uterine tissue producing a negative nitrogen balance. The shrinkage is known as involution. The fundal height is checked to detect any delay in involution (*Fig.* 15.1).

246

The hypertrophied spiral arteries and veins of the placental bed become thrombosed soon after delivery and degenerate. The uterus continues to contract regularly in the puerperium and expels debris of cast-off decidua. The contractions may be so strong as to give rise to pain, particularly in the multigravida. These 'after-pains' are especially noted during suckling, and the mother may require mild analgesics in the first few days.

Lochia

Lochia (from Gk. *lochos,* childbirth) is the name given to the discharge from the uterus which lasts for 3–6 weeks after delivery. For the first few days the discharge is mainly blood, then for the next 7–10 days it is a paler serosanguinous loss and becomes yellowish for up to 6 weeks. The lochia consists of red blood cells, leucocytes, decidual cells and fibrinous products. The bacterial flora normally found in the vagina return within 72 hours and may include anaerobic streptococci, *E.coli,* staphylococci and *Clostridium welchii.* A mixed growth of such organisms is not evidence of infection of the genital tract. When infection occurs it causes clinical signs (*see below*). Lochia from the uterus is alkaline. It becomes acid in the vagina and its constituents decompose due to the action of bacterial saprophytes. If lochia is retained it becomes offensive.

Prevention of Ascending Genital Tract Infection

The patient should be in a clean environment. The room, furnishings and linen should all be clean, as should the patient, all attendants and visitors. Masks should be worn whenever the vulva is exposed and strict aseptic techniques should be used if a vaginal examination is done. The care of the vulva can usually be undertaken by the patient herself. Frequent showers and regular use of a bidet have superseded vulval swabbings. Special attention should be paid to vulval toilet after defaecation, avoiding drawing anal organisms forward over the vulva. The temperature is taken twice daily, and the lochia is observed, a note being made of the amount (increased loss suggests retained placenta or membranes) and colour. Offensive lochia and pyrexia suggest infection.

The Perineum

Lacerations or an episiotomy should be inspected daily to note healing and sutures are removed on day 5 or 6 by which time skin healing should have occurred. Complete deep tissue healing occurs in 3 weeks. The pain from a bruised or swollen perineum may be relieved by ice packs, local anaesthetic sprays (beware allergic reactions!) and mild analgesics. Ultrasound may also be helpful in reducing oedema and bruising. The contact medium used is water, as the usual liquid paraffin is obviously unsuitable for the damaged perineum. The patient lies in a bath. The transducer head is held as close as possible and moved slowly over the perineum, but direct contact is avoided.

In diagnostic ultrasound 20 mW per cm^2 is used. For this purpose 0·5 W per cm^2 for 5 minutes twice daily is used, and the perineum reviewed after 3 days. In cases of severe damage the treatment has to be continued for a further 2 or 3 days.

The cervical os admits 1—2 fingers for 7—10 days after delivery. The external os never regains its nulliparous appearance, being stretched or lacerated to some extent in labour (*Fig.* 15.2).

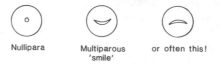

Nullipara   Multiparous   or often this!
                 'smile'

Fig. 15.2. Appearance of external os.

The pouting endocervical epithelium so commonly seen on the ecto-cervix during pregnancy under the misnomer of 'erosion of pregnancy' gradually disappears during the puerperium and has usually gone by 6 weeks.

The vagina slowly shrinks and rugae reappear in the third week.

Ovarian Function

This gradually returns as prolactin levels fall, stimulating regeneration of the endometrium and formation of new spiral vessels, some by recanaliz-ation within the thrombosed lumens of old vessels. Regeneration of the endometrium usually takes 6 weeks, although very occasionally pregnancy may occur before this time indicating a more rapid return of ovarian function.

Urinary Tract

Micturition should occur within 12 hours of delivery and by day 2 a diuresis has occurred and most of the fluid retained during pregnancy is excreted. The changes in glomerular filtration revert rapidly to normal, but the dilatation of the ureters seen in pregnancy does not disappear until 12 or more weeks after delivery. Urinary tract infection is very common, especially if the patient has been catheterized in labour. Acute retention, and retention with overflow may occur, especially following operative vaginal delivery. These complications are often limited to the first 24—48 hours. If overlooked, permanent damage to the kidneys and bladder may occur. Catheterization is required and may need to be repeated. If the patient is still unable to micturate then bladder drainage with an indwelling catheter is required. If the patient is catheterized, frequent bacteriological examination of the urine is necessary and prompt treatment with anti-biotics is needed if infection develops. Should continuous urinary incontinence be noticed then a fistula must be sought. This is extremely rare in this country but is more common after prolonged obstructed labour, difficult intravaginal manoeuvres or inexpertly executed Caesarean section.

Blood

The haemoglobin level is stable by day 5, as the increased blood volume disappears with the early postpartum diuresis. The leucocytosis of pregnancy (which may reach 30 000 cells per mm^3 in labour) falls to 10 000 cells per mm^3 by day 4. The platelet count increases by day 4 and rises to a maximum by day 10. There is an increase in platelet 'stickiness' and immature platelet forms are seen in the blood film. These changes, together with increased fibrinogen, explain the liability to puerperal thromboembolism. The changes in the clotting factors during pregnancy gradually revert to normal.

Gastrointestinal Tract

Defaecation should occur by the third day, but there is a tendency to constipation which is enhanced by the lack of exercise, fluid loss, restriction of food intake during labour and fear of pain if the perineum is sore. Constipation is often a source of concern to the patient. Fruit, fluids and bran are to be encouraged, but a mild laxative may be needed. Analgesic suppositories and cream will ease haemorrhoids which will improve during the puerperium. The patient should eat whatever she wishes, but if she is lactating at least 2 litres of fluid are necessary.

Metabolism

There is an increase in urinary nitrogen due to intense muscle breakdown, and peptones are present for the first 10 days. It is not unusual to find lactose and traces of albumin during this time. The basal metabolic rate returns to normal and a glucose tolerance test returns to normal within 48 hours.

Psychology

Minor emotional disturbances are very common, the elation of the first 48 hours classically giving way to the depression of the 'fourth day blues'. These changes gradually settle over the next few days. Although insomnia, excessive mood change and depression may be premonitory signs of puerperal psychosis in the immediate puerperium, the manifestations may not be apparent until some weeks after delivery. Poor bonding, inadequate care of the child and loss of interest may also be early signs. Depression is the main feature and if not detected early and treated promptly may lead to major disability, family breakdown, infanticide and suicide. Most psychiatric hospitals have special mother and baby units for patients with puerperal psychosis so that the mother is not separated from her baby yet is supervised while with it.

OBJECTIVES OF CARE IN THE PUERPERIUM

Briefly the objectives of care may be summarized as:

1. to establish bonding;
2. to establish or suppress lactation;
3. to prevent or detect early bleeding, sepsis or thromboembolism.

Bonding

An intimate psychological unity between mother and infant can be achieved in the hours and days after delivery. Such a relationship has profound beneficial effects on the child, especially during its formative years, and for the mother. The opportunity for creating this bonding exists only in the immediate puerperium and should anything interfere with its establishment then the bonding will be at best inadequate, at worst non-existent.

The mother and baby should be together as much as possible. She should hold the baby at the time of delivery if this is feasible and continue to hold the baby, under supervision if necessary, for as long as she wishes. The baby should be put to the breast if she has decided to breast-feed as soon as it is convenient for her to do so. If the father is present he should be encouraged to handle the child, with his wife, and other children should be introduced to their new sibling at the earliest appropriate time. The re-establishment of the family unit is of major importance but should not interfere with the bonding of mother and new offspring.

Ideally the mother and baby should only be separated at the wishes of the mother, but if, for medical reasons, the infant is taken into a special care unit then free and frequent access is to be encouraged. If the mother is ill the baby should be brought to her as often as her condition permits. Any separation should be bridged by the father and other offspring as appropriate. The young primipara may need encouragement and guidance to establish her confidence but ideally she and the father will have been prepared during antenatal parentcraft classes.

Lactation (*See* Chapter 12 for physiology of lactation)

The decision about how to feed the baby is the mother's, but the decision should be made during the antenatal period after full and free discussion and in the knowledge of the facts about breast- and bottle-feeding. The mother who decides she does not wish to breast-feed or finds she does not lactate should not be made to feel guilty. She will need as much assistance and supervision during the early days while bottle-feeding as the mother who breast-feeds.

Breast milk is instantly available, of the right consistency and content, at the ideal temperature and is free. Also, of great importance, it contains high levels of antibodies – as does colostrum, the pre-milk flow. (Milk 'comes in' about the third day.) The arguments that 'I'll be slower to get my figure back', 'It ties me down as only I can do it', and 'It takes too long to learn' are fatuous.

Bottle-feeding is perhaps slightly faster because the teat is bigger. It is, however, expensive, requires lengthy preparation, and carries the hazards of protein allergy, excessive salt ingestion and infection. This last is due to poor sterilization and the lack of antibodies. Also it interferes with bonding.

Feeding

When she feeds her baby the mother should be relaxed with no other concern. She should be settled wherever she is most comfortable; this is usually in or on the bed, or in a low chair which gives good support. She may find a footstool comfortable. Some mothers enjoy the closer contact obtained by baring the top half of the body and the baby undressed except for a nappy and shawl.

The mother should support the baby's head and ensure that the nose is clear of her body as the newborn baby is unable to breathe through its mouth. She should see that the baby's tongue is depressed, and, if breast-feeding, that the baby 'fixes' on the breast, so that the whole nipple and most of the areola is taken into the baby's mouth. If bottle-feeding then the entire end of the teat is taken into the mouth over the depressed tongue.

Feeding is not instinctive; it has to be learned by the mother and child, and it is essential that guidance and help is readily available during the learning time. The baby should be fed when it is hungry and for as long as it is hungry. The baby should not be allowed to remain on the breast for excessive lengths of time as soreness and cracking of the nipples may result. Most babies eventually establish a routine but the rigid '2 minutes on each breast initially increasing through 5 and 10 to 15 minutes each side every 4 hours' does not suit every mother and baby, and if imposed may cause feeding problems and the mother may give up breast-feeding. A nursing brassiere which gives good support provides comfort. The application of a little lanolin cream to the nipples will prevent excessive drying.

Difficult lactation is often due to poor motivation, but occasionally is due to general ill health. Inverted nipples and sore cracked nipples may lead to difficult lactation. If the engorged breast does not have some milk expressed before feeding, or if the breast is not emptied at feeding and the remaining milk not expressed then lactation will subside.

Suppression of lactation is most satisfactorily achieved by avoiding stimulation of the nipples and firmly binding the breasts. Mild analgesics may be required about the third day because as the milk comes in the breasts become engorged and very tender. Should it be necessary to suppress established lactation then bromocriptine, which suppresses prolactin, is to be preferred to oestrogens because of the risk of thromboembolism. The dose regime is bromocriptine 2·5 mg initially then 2·5 mg b.d. for 14 days.

Prevention and Detection of the Major Puerperal Complications

The major puerperal complications are bleeding, sepsis and thrombo-embolism.

Bleeding

The first hour following delivery and primary postpartum haemorrhage is included under management of labour (*see* Chapter 14). Careful observation of the uterus, vaginal loss and mother's pulse and blood pressure should be made regularly during the first 4 hours to detect evidence of excessive bleeding. If that occurs it is often due to clots in the uterus or vagina. Massage of the uterus and expression of the clots, together with an injection of ergometrine and further observation is indicated. If further bleeding occurs the vagina and uterus should be explored under general anaesthesia.

Secondary PPH

This is defined as excessive·blood loss from the genital tract after the first 24 hours following delivery. No precise volume is specified.

If bleeding occurs in the first few days after delivery it is likely to be due to retained fragments of placenta, retained membranes or blood clot. Bleeding occurring later may be due to infection of the endometrium or to impaired involution of the spiral vessels or abnormal regeneration of these vessels. Infection may, however, occur in retained products.

On examination the uterus is larger than expected, is usually tender, and the os may be open. The blood may be offensive and the mother pyrexial. Evacuation of the uterus should be done in all such cases under general anaesthesia. It is easy to damage the uterus. A high vaginal swab should always be taken, and if there is any clinical suspicion of infection systemic antibiotics started before the culture result is available. If there is no evidence of infection and the bleeding is slight the patient may be kept under observation. Ergometrine is of dubious use here, but if bleeding is heavier or continuous the uterus must be explored and parenteral ergometrine (0·5 mg ergometrine intramuscularly) may be given.

Sepsis

In past centuries childbed fever has carried millions of women to their graves but it is now an uncommon cause of maternal death.

Definition of Puerperal Pyrexia ʃₐₜ. 38°C. 24hr., 2/d.

England and Wales: 'Any febrile condition occurring in a woman in whom a temperature of 38 °C or more has occurred within 14 days after confinement or miscarriage'.

Causes of Puerperal Pyrexia

1. Genital tract infection. The sign is a tender bulky uterus. (Occasionally perineal infection may cause pyrexia without involving the upper genital tract.)

2. Urinary tract infection.
3. Deep venous thrombosis.
4. Mastitis. The sign is a tender red area.
5. Respiratory infection, especially after anaesthesia.
6. Unrelated causes (e.g. appendicitis).

Management of Puerperal Pyrexia

1. Detailed history.
2. General physical examination.
3. Isolate the mother and baby.
4. Look for the cause of the pyrexia before instituting therapy by microscopy and culture of:

> high vaginal swab;
> clean specimen of urine;
> throat swab;
> (blood for culture).

5. Prompt prescription of a broad-spectrum antibiotic (e.g. ampicillin 500 mg orally 6-hourly) when genitourinary infection seems the likely cause. The addition of an agent such as metronidazole which is effective against anaerobic organisms in doses of 400 mg orally thrice daily is becoming standard practice.

Genital Tract Infection

The patient is particularly vulnerable to ascending genital tract infections during the early puerperium, and every effort must be made as described earlier in this chapter to prevent infection. The placental site can be likened to a wound and the perineum and/or vagina may be damaged by laceration or episiotomy.

The natural defence mechanisms of the vagina and cervix have been destroyed by pregnancy and delivery. The uterus contains a great deal of cellular debris and small pieces of necrotic tissue in a relatively anaerobic atmosphere, an ideal environment for the growth of organisms. Infection is particularly common after prolonged labour and prolonged rupture of the membranes. The effects are aggravated by anaemia and ill health. *Fig.* 15.3 shows the pathways of spread of infection.

Clinically the patient may feel unwell, complain of pain and tenderness in the lower abdomen and of offensive lochia which may become a deeper red and heavier. On examination she may be found to be pyrexial with a tender uterus.

PATHOGENS

β-haemolytic streptococci caused major outbreaks of puerperal fever in the past. The organisms responsible may come from the patient or more usually her attendants. Commensals from the rectum, nose, hands etc., such as coliforms, *Streptococcus faecalis,* clostridium, staphylococci and streptococci may all be implicated.

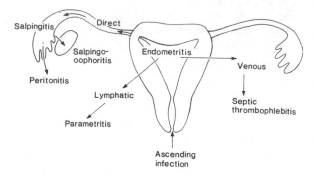

Fig. 15.3. Pathways of spread of genital infection.

MANAGEMENT
The priorities are:

appropriate antibiotic therapy;
adequate analgesia;
rest;
adequate hydration.

The sequelae of sterility, chronic ill health or death should be avoided by early detection and prompt treatment.

Thromboembolism
This continues to be one of the most frequent causes of maternal death.

Prevention
Early ambulation is to be encouraged, particularly after Caesarean section or operative vaginal delivery when the risks of thromboembolism are greatest. The patient should be instructed to carry out leg movements and start a course of postnatal exercises to help reduce the risks of thrombo-embolism and restore muscle tone. Prophylactic anticoagulants should be used in selected cases, and oestrogens to suppress lactation should be avoided.

Management
It is important to establish a firm diagnosis promptly (venogram or radio-active iodine studies), since the diagnosis has implications for the patient's future (e.g. further pregnancies and operations, and oral contraception). Initial treatment is with heparin and subsequently with oral anticoagulants for 6 weeks.

Further Reading

Morgan G. (1978) Psychiatric disorders. In: Browne J. C. McC. and Dixon H. G. (ed.), *Browne's Antenatal Care*, 11th ed. Edinburgh, Churchill Livingstone.

Report on Confidential Enquiries into Maternal Deaths in England and Wales 1973–1975. (1979) London, HMSO.

Stanway P. and Stanway A. (1978) *Breast is Best.* London, Pan.

Tindall V. R. (1978) Venous thrombosis. In: Macdonald R. R. (ed.) *Scientific Basis of Obstetrics and Gynaecology.* Edinburgh, Churchill Livingstone.

Chapter sixteen
Maternal and Perinatal Mortality

It is difficult to realize that at the turn of this century 5 mothers in every 1000 died in childbirth, and it is not uncommon for the grandparents of the present generation to have known at least one person who died having a baby. With improving health and nutrition and a general increase in the standard of living as the twentieth century advanced, the number of mothers dying in childbirth decreased and continues to do so. Certainly the advent of antibiotics and blood transfusion played a part, and it is tempting for obstetricians to ascribe a major role to the development of antenatal care, but the most important factor has been the rising socio-economic status and general health of the population.

In the last half of this century the series of Reports on Confidential Enquiries into Maternal Deaths in England and Wales (there are similar separate Reports for Scotland) has also contributed to the fall in maternal mortality (*see Fig.* 16.1). A maternal death in the Reports is defined as 'one occurring during the pregnancy or during labour or as a consequence of pregnancy, within one year of delivery or abortion'. The Area Medical Officer issues an enquiry form which is filled in by all persons involved with the patient during her pregnancy: the general practitioner, community midwife, hospital consultant and medical staff of all grades and specialties and hospital midwives. These forms are confidential, being collected and analysed by the Department of Health and Social Security's advisers in obstetrics and gynaecology and anaesthetics, with help from the Medical Statistics Unit of the Office of Population Censuses and Surveys. The analyses, in which patients and localities are anonymous, are published ever 3 years, the first Report covering the years 1952—1954 and the most recent 1973—1975. The Reports list 'avoidable factors', that is where 'there was departure from generally accepted standards of satisfactory care', and relate instances (anonymously) and highlight particular problems. For instance, as a result of the earlier Reports it became apparent that it was unwise to transfer a patient with a retained placenta after delivery at home as she was frequently moribund on arrival at the major unit. The Report's recommendations that obstetric flying squads should be called to such cases were followed by a reduction in mortality from this cause. The

Reports pointed out the frequency of maternal deaths due to anaesthetic causes where the anaesthetist was a junior, and consequently a major reorganization of obstetric anaesthetic services has occurred.

The main causes of true maternal death, that is those directly due to pregnancy or delivery are, in order of frequency in the latest 1973–1975 Report: (1) hypertensive diseases of pregnancy (H), (2) pulmonary embolism (E), (3) abortion (A) and (4) haemorrhage (B) (nemonic – HEAB). These have been the major causes of death since the first 1952–1954 Report, but the order has varied and for each cause the numbers have decreased, in spite of fluctuations in the number of births.

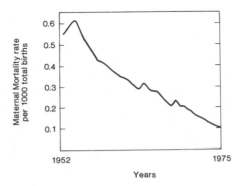

Fig. 16.1. Maternal mortality (excluding abortion) rate per 1000 total births 1952–1975. Data from Report on Confidential Enquiries into Maternal Deaths in England and Wales 1973–75.

It is sad to see such a high percentage of avoidable factors in each group in all the Reports. The most frequent avoidable factor is neglect of the basic principles of antenatal care by consultant obstetricians and general practitioners. This is stressed repeatedly for each major cause of maternal death, especially the hypertensive diseases of pregnancy. Although the number of deaths from haemorrhage are fewer in the latest Report, the mortality rate for this cause has remained the same for the last two Reports. The latest Report indeed emphasizes yet again the need to call the flying squad when a patient has a severe haemorrhage at home and states that early and adequate blood transfusion is essential.

The number of deaths from pulmonary embolism during pregnancy was the same in the last two Reports, but as the number of births has fallen the actual incidence of such deaths has increased. The latest Report points out that maternal obesity and bed rest for hypertension or fetal growth retardation are predisposing factors, that the risk of thromboembolism increases with age, parity and operative procedures, especially Caesarean section, and reiterates the advice that caution be exercised before suppressing lactation with oestrogens.

The maternal mortality rate (excluding abortion) for the years 1973–1975 was 11·35 per 100 000 total births. All the Reports show considerable differences between maternal mortality rates in different regions. The highest rate is 18·64 in the North-East Thames region and the lowest is 4·38 in the Oxford region. Every student of obstetrics should peruse these reports carefully. The number of avoidable factors must be reduced to bring about a further decrease in maternal mortality.

The term 'Perinatal Mortality Rate' means stillbirths plus first-week deaths per 1000 total births and is a combination of the stillbirth rate and the neonatal death rate. The stillbirth rate is the number of stillborn infants per 1000 total births and the neonatal death rate is the number of first-week deaths per 1000 live births. As with maternal deaths there has been a dramatic fall in perinatal mortality during this century, due largely to the improving health of the obstetric population (see Fig. 16.2). It is difficult for the present generation to believe that in the poverty-stricken South Wales mining villages in the 1850s the perinatal and infant mortality rate was nearly 50 per cent, in other words a pregnant woman had only a 50–50 chance of having an infant still alive a year after delivery. The decline in perinatal mortality in England and Wales since World War II is also due to the results of three major surveys. The first figures of perinatal mortality in England and Wales came from the year 1946 when the first National Maternity Survey was made. The British perinatal mortality survey published its first report in 1963 and this was based on a national sample of 17 000 births which occurred in one week of 1958. There is an additional sample of 7000 perinatal deaths occurring over 3 months. The design of this report was unique and the information obtained had a profound effect on obstetric and paediatric practice, leading to many improvements in maternity services. A second report based on the same national sample was published in 1969, defining and analysing in detail high-risk pregnancies. Because of the great value of the information obtained and the subsequent improvement of maternal and neonatal care a further survey (British Births 1970) looking at all deliveries which took place during one week in 1970 was executed. As can be seen in Fig. 16.2, the perinatal mortality rate has continued to decline, being 23·7 per 1000 total births in 1970 and about 18·0 in 1979. However, if one looks at the international scene, making allowances for differences in culture and wealth, the UK comes somewhere in the middle and is in fact tending to slide down the scale. This suggests that further improvements in perinatal care are possible and must be incorporated into obstetric and neonatal services here, as they have been in many other countries.

We will use the results of the survey British Births 1970 to illustrate the main causes of perinatal deaths. In the survey there were 395 stillbirths and first-week deaths giving a perinatal mortality rate of 23·7 per 1000 births. Although the rate is now lower the causes of death remain the same and in approximately the same ratios. Stillbirths accounted for 54 per cent of perinatal deaths. Half of these stillbirths showed changes due to severe intrauterine anoxia, and major congenital malformation was found in 20 per cent. Common lesions were anencephalus, hydrocephalus with spina bifida and meningomyelocele and gross cardiac malformation. Rhesus incompatibility gave rise to 7 cases of hydrops fetalis and there were 2 cases of birth trauma.

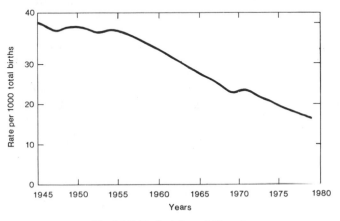

Fig. 16.2. Perinatal mortality rate.

There were 180 neonatal deaths, just under half of the total (46 per cent). The major cause of neonatal death was hyaline membrane disease and respiratory distress syndrome (RDS), which accounted for 30 per cent of deaths. Congenital malformations accounted for nearly a quarter of the deaths (23 per cent), anoxia 17 per cent and gross immaturity, that is very small infants under 1000 g at birth, 15 per cent. Infection and birth trauma were less common causes, accounting for 2 and 3 per cent of neonatal deaths respectively.

It is interesting that deaths from respiratory distress syndrome were more common in males, being 3 : 1 male preponderance, and 84 per cent of these babies dying from RDS were under 2500 g and delivered prematurely. In nearly half of these cases there was a maternal factor, either hypertensive disease or antepartum haemorrhage, which was responsible for the premature delivery, but no such cause could be found for the rest.

In the survey there were 39 cases of congenital malformations in singletons, accounting for 24 per cent of neonatal deaths; 22 of these infants weighed less than 2500 g and the male to female ratio was 3 : 2. Individual malformations vary in their sex incidence, and anencephalus is more common in the female.

Anoxia and birth trauma are considered together since anoxia predisposes to birth trauma. An instrumental delivery may be necessary if anoxia develops antepartum, and such a delivery may cause intracranial haemorrhage leading to a stillbirth or neonatal death. In this survey anoxia was thought to be the main case of death in 30 neonates (8·3 per cent). There were 4 cases of undoubted birth trauma causing neonatal death and 2 more cases causing stillbirths.

Immaturity, that is excessively small infants under 1000 g, accounted for nearly 5 per cent of neonatal deaths. Haemolytic disease caused 7 stillbirths and 4 first-week deaths, and infection 4 deaths.

It is important to remember that although a death is a readily recordable event and therefore death rates are used as the measure of achievement, an equal, if not greater, concern must be expressed about perinatal morbidity and the quality of life of survivors. This is a much more. difficult area where precise analysis and statistics are not possible. Perinatal mortality may be likened to the tip of an iceberg with neonatal morbidity lying beneath unseen.

It is hoped that a reduction in perinatal mortality will result in a diminution of perinatal morbidity since some causes of death also cause defects in survivors.

Mothers	Major Causes of Death Stillbirths	Neonates
Hypertensive diseases	Anoxia	Respiratory distress syndrome
Pulmonary embolism	Congenital malformations	Congenital malformations
Abortion		Anoxia
		Gross immaturity <1000 g
Haemorrhage	Rhesus incompatibility	

Further Reading
British Births 1970, vol. 1. (1975) London, Heinemann.
Butler N. R. and Bonham D. G. (1963) *Perinatal Mortality*. Edinburgh, E. & S. Livingstone.
Report on Confidential Enquiries into Maternal Deaths in England and Wales 1973–1975. (1975) London, HMSO.

Index